ZONE DIET

Achieve Optimal Health and Weight Loss with Balanced Nutrition

Charles M. Calvert

CONTENTS

PREFACE

Welcome to the world of the "Zone Diet"!

In a time when diet trends come and go, it can be overwhelming to navigate through the sea of information. The Zone Diet, however, has withstood the test of time and continues to be a powerful approach to achieving optimal health and wellness.

This book serves as your guide to understanding and implementing the principles of the Zone Diet. Whether you are new to the concept or looking to refresh your knowledge, these pages will equip you with the tools and insights to make informed choices about your nutrition.

The Zone Diet, developed by Dr. Barry Sears, is a balanced and scientifically-backed approach to eating that focuses on maintaining a state of hormonal balance. By carefully balancing the ratio of macronutrients—carbohydrates, proteins, and fats—we can support our body's metabolic processes, control inflammation, and optimize overall well-being.

Throughout this book, you will discover the fundamental principles of the Zone Diet, along with practical strategies for incorporating them into your daily life. From understanding the importance of the "Zone" ratio to learning about the power of anti-inflammatory foods, each chapter is designed to empower you to take control of your nutrition and improve your health.

As you embark on your journey with the Zone Diet, remember that it is not just a temporary solution but a sustainable and lifelong approach to nutrition. Embrace the concept of balance, and be patient with yourself as you navigate the path to achieving your health goals. The Zone Diet is not about deprivation or strict rules; it is about nourishing your body and finding harmony within.

I hope that this book will serve as a valuable resource, guiding you towards a healthier and more balanced life. May it empower you to make informed choices about your nutrition, inspire you to embrace a lifelong commitment to your well-being, and ultimately contribute to your overall health and happiness.

Wishing you success on your journey to discovering the power of the Zone Diet!

INTRODUCTION

Importance Of Maintaining A Healthy Weight And Energy Levels

Maintaining a healthy weight and energy levels is crucial for overall well-being and optimal functioning of the body. It not only enhances physical appearance but also plays a significant role in preventing various health issues and improving quality of life. In this article, we will explore the importance of maintaining a healthy weight and energy levels and the positive impact it can have on overall health.

1. Physical Health Benefits

One of the primary reasons to maintain a healthy weight and energy levels is to reduce the risk of developing chronic diseases such as heart disease, diabetes, and certain types of cancer. Excess weight puts additional strain on the cardiovascular system and can lead to high blood pressure and elevated cholesterol levels. By maintaining a healthy weight, you can lower the risk of these conditions and promote a healthy heart.

Moreover, maintaining a healthy weight helps to keep the body's blood sugar levels stable, reducing the risk of developing type 2 diabetes. It also decreases the likelihood of developing joint problems and conditions like osteoarthritis, as excess weight puts extra stress on the joints.

2. Mental Well-being

In addition to the physical benefits, maintaining a healthy weight and energy levels positively impacts mental well-being. Regular exercise, which is an essential component of weight maintenance, releases endorphins that help elevate mood and reduce stress. It can also improve sleep quality, leading to increased energy levels during the day and improved cognitive function.

Furthermore, individuals who maintain a healthy weight often report higher self-esteem and body confidence. This can have a profound impact on mental health, promoting a positive body image and reducing the risk of developing eating disorders or body dysmorphia.

3. Increased Energy Levels

Maintaining a healthy weight is closely linked to sustaining optimal energy levels throughout the day. When we consume a well-balanced diet that provides all the necessary nutrients, our bodies are fueled adequately to perform daily activities efficiently. Proper nutrition, combined with regular exercise, helps improve blood circulation and oxygen delivery to the muscles, resulting in increased energy levels.

Moreover, excess weight can lead to feelings of fatigue and sluggishness due to the additional strain placed on the body's systems. By maintaining a healthy weight, the body functions more efficiently, reducing the burden on the cardiovascular system and allowing for better circulation and oxygenation of tissues.

4. Longevity and Quality of Life

Maintaining a healthy weight and energy levels is strongly associated with increased longevity and improved quality of life. By avoiding the risks associated with obesity and sedentary lifestyles, individuals can enjoy a more active and fulfilling life. A healthy weight contributes to better mobility, making it easier to engage in physical activities and enjoy hobbies.

Additionally, by maintaining a healthy weight, individuals often experience fewer health complications, resulting in a lower reliance on medication and healthcare services. This can lead to reduced healthcare costs and an improved overall sense of well-being.

Overview Of "The Zone" Program

"The Zone" program is a dietary approach that focuses on balancing macronutrients in meals to stabilize blood sugar levels, control hunger, and optimize overall health. Developed by Dr. Barry Sears, the program gained popularity in the 1990s and continues to be followed by many individuals seeking weight loss and improved well-being. In this section, we will provide an overview of "The Zone" program and its key principles.

1. The Zone Ratio

The Zone program emphasizes a specific macronutrient ratio in each meal, which is 40% carbohydrates, 30% protein, and 30% fat. This ratio aims to balance insulin levels and control inflammation in the body. By adhering to this ratio, individuals can maintain stable blood sugar levels, reduce cravings, and achieve optimal hormonal balance.

2. Controlling Insulin Levels

Insulin is a hormone responsible for regulating blood sugar levels. When blood sugar spikes after a meal, the body releases insulin to transport the glucose into cells for energy or storage. However, excessive insulin production can lead to fat storage and energy crashes. "The Zone" program focuses on controlling insulin levels by consuming meals that maintain a steady blood sugar response.

3. The Importance of Protein

Protein plays a significant role in "The Zone" program. It helps to stabilize blood sugar levels, control hunger, and support muscle growth and repair. By including a sufficient amount of protein in each meal, individuals can feel fuller for longer periods and maintain stable energy levels throughout the day.

4. Balancing Omega-3 and Omega-6 Fatty Acids

"The Zone" program emphasizes the consumption of healthy fats, particularly those rich in omega-3 fatty acids. Omega-3 fatty acids are known for their anti-inflammatory properties, while omega-6 fatty acids can promote inflammation when consumed in excess. Balancing the intake of these two types of fats is believed to reduce inflammation in the body and support overall health.

5. The Importance of Meal Timing

Another key principle of "The Zone" program is meal timing. The program recommends eating every four to five hours to maintain stable blood sugar levels and avoid energy crashes. By spacing out meals in this way, individuals can regulate hunger, prevent overeating, and keep their metabolism active throughout the day.

6. Personalized Approach

"The Zone" program acknowledges that individual requirements may vary, and it encourages a personalized approach. Factors such as body composition, activity levels, and overall health are taken into consideration when determining the appropriate portion sizes and macronutrient ratios for each person. This personalized approach ensures that individuals can adapt the program to suit their specific needs and goals.

Purpose Of The Ebook

The purpose of the ebook is to offer readers a comprehensive guide to eating well, losing weight, and increasing energy levels. It aims to provide valuable information, practical tips, and actionable strategies that individuals can implement in their daily lives to achieve their health and wellness goals. In this section, we will delve into the main objectives and content that the ebook covers.

1. Educating Readers on Proper Nutrition

The ebook seeks to educate readers about the fundamentals of proper nutrition. It covers essential topics such as macronutrients (carbohydrates, proteins, and fats), micronutrients (vitamins and minerals), and the importance of a balanced diet. By providing a clear understanding of nutrition principles, the ebook empowers readers to make informed decisions about their food choices.

2. Weight Loss Strategies

A significant focus of the ebook is on weight loss strategies. It provides evidence-based approaches to achieving and maintaining a healthy weight. This includes information on creating a calorie deficit, portion control, mindful eating, and incorporating regular physical activity. The ebook explores various dietary patterns and offers guidance on finding a weight loss approach that suits individual preferences and lifestyles.

3. Meal Planning and Recipes

To support readers in their journey towards eating well, the ebook includes practical tips and strategies for meal planning. It provides guidance on creating balanced meals, incorporating a variety of nutrients, and making healthy food choices. Additionally, the ebook may offer a selection of delicious and nutritious recipes to inspire readers and help them explore new flavors and culinary options.

4. Boosting Energy Levels

The ebook recognizes the importance of maintaining optimal energy levels. It may provide insights on the role of proper nutrition, regular exercise, quality sleep, and stress management in promoting sustained energy throughout the day. The ebook may offer practical suggestions on incorporating energy-boosting foods, staying hydrated, and adopting lifestyle habits that enhance overall vitality.

5. Behavior Change and Mindset

Understanding that long-term success in eating well and achieving weight loss requires a positive mindset and sustainable behavior change, the ebook may dedicate sections to address these aspects. It may provide guidance on setting realistic goals, developing healthy habits, managing cravings, and overcoming common barriers to success. By focusing on mindset and behavior, the ebook aims to support readers in making lasting changes and maintaining their progress.

6. Additional Topics

Depending on the scope of the ebook, it may cover additional topics related to nutrition and wellness. These could include discussions on the role of supplements, the impact of hydration on health, the benefits of mindful eating, tips for eating out or traveling, and strategies for maintaining a healthy lifestyle in the long term. The goal is to provide a comprehensive resource that covers various aspects of eating well, weight loss, and increasing energy levels.

CHAPTER ONE

Understanding The Zone

What Is The Zone Diet?

The Zone diet is a popular dietary approach that was developed by Dr. Barry Sears, a biochemist and author, in the mid-1990s. It is a balanced eating plan that aims to regulate the body's hormone levels by controlling the intake of macronutrients, namely carbohydrates, proteins, and fats. The main premise of The Zone diet is to maintain a specific ratio of these macronutrients in each meal, which is 40% carbohydrates, 30% protein, and 30% fat.

The concept behind The Zone diet is based on the idea that consuming the right balance of macronutrients helps to stabilize blood sugar levels, control inflammation, and optimize hormonal balance. By adhering to this ratio, it is believed that individuals can achieve a state called "the zone," where the body operates at its peak performance.

Explanation Of The Concept And Principles Behind The Zone

The principles of The Zone diet revolve around the impact of macronutrients on hormone regulation and inflammation. According to Dr. Sears, the ratio of 40:30:30 (carbohydrates:protein:fat) helps to control the production of insulin, a hormone that regulates blood sugar levels. By keeping insulin levels in check, it is believed that the body can burn fat more efficiently and maintain stable energy levels throughout the day.

One of the key concepts in The Zone diet is the concept of the "block." A block is a unit of measurement used to determine the quantity of food consumed in each meal. A typical block consists of a specific amount of protein, carbohydrate, and fat. The exact measurements vary based on an individual's body size and activity level, but the overall goal is to maintain the 40:30:30 ratio.

To determine the number of blocks required per day, individuals need to consider their body composition, activity level, and goals. The Zone diet typically recommends consuming a certain number of blocks per day, spread evenly across meals and snacks. By carefully balancing the macronutrients in each block, the diet aims to regulate hormonal responses and control inflammation in the body.

Benefits Of Following The Zone Diet

1. **Stable blood sugar levels**: The Zone diet focuses on controlling insulin levels, which can lead to stable blood sugar levels throughout the day. This may help prevent energy crashes and reduce cravings for sugary or high-carbohydrate foods.

2. **Weight management**: By regulating insulin and promoting fat burning, The Zone diet may support weight loss and weight maintenance. The balanced macronutrient ratio and portion control can help individuals feel satisfied while maintaining a calorie deficit, which is essential for weight management.

3. **Improved hormonal balance**: The Zone diet aims to optimize hormonal balance by controlling the release of insulin. This can have positive effects on other hormones, such as glucagon, which promotes fat breakdown, and eicosanoids, which regulate inflammation.

4. **Reduced inflammation**: Chronic inflammation is associated with various health issues, including heart disease, diabetes, and autoimmune conditions. The Zone diet emphasizes anti-inflammatory foods, such as fruits, vegetables, and healthy fats, which may help reduce inflammation in the body.

5. **Enhanced athletic performance**: Some proponents of The Zone diet believe that it can improve athletic performance by providing a steady supply of energy and supporting muscle recovery. The balanced macronutrient ratio may help optimize nutrient absorption and utilization during exercise.

6. **Healthier eating habits**: The Zone diet encourages individuals to focus on whole, unprocessed foods and to pay attention to portion sizes. This can lead to a shift towards a healthier and more mindful approach to eating, promoting long-term sustainable habits.

7. **Improved cardiovascular health**: The Zone diet promotes the consumption of lean proteins, healthy fats, and low-glycemic carbohydrates, which can have a positive impact on cardiovascular health. By controlling insulin levels and reducing inflammation, it may help lower the risk of heart disease and improve lipid profiles.

8. **Flexibility and customization**: While The Zone diet emphasizes specific macronutrient ratios, it allows for flexibility in food choices. It encourages the inclusion of a wide variety of fruits, vegetables, lean proteins, healthy fats, and whole grains. This flexibility makes it easier to customize meals according to personal preferences and dietary restrictions.

9. **Long-term sustainability**: The balanced approach of The Zone diet, combined with its emphasis on whole foods and portion control, can contribute to long-term sustainability. Rather than relying on drastic restrictions or fad diets, The Zone diet promotes a balanced and moderate eating plan that can be maintained over the long term.

The Hormonal Balance Theory

The hormonal balance theory is a concept that suggests hormones play a crucial role in maintaining overall health and well-being. Hormones are chemical messengers produced by various glands in the body that regulate numerous bodily functions, including growth, metabolism, mood, and reproduction. According to this theory, maintaining a delicate balance of hormones is essential for optimal physical and mental health.

1. Key Hormones: Several hormones are involved in the body's complex regulatory system. Some of the key hormones include:

- **Estrogen and Progesterone:** These are primary female sex hormones responsible for menstrual cycle regulation, fertility, and the development of secondary sexual characteristics.

- **Testosterone:** The primary male sex hormone that influences muscle mass, bone density, libido, and overall vitality.

- **Insulin:** Produced by the pancreas, insulin regulates blood sugar levels and facilitates the absorption of glucose into cells.

- **Cortisol:** Released by the adrenal glands, cortisol helps the body respond to stress, regulates metabolism, and influences immune function.

- **Thyroid Hormones:** Triiodothyronine (T3) and thyroxine (T4) are produced by the thyroid gland and regulate metabolism, growth, and development.

2. Hormonal Imbalances: When the delicate balance of hormones is disrupted, it can lead to various health issues. Hormonal imbalances can occur due to factors such as stress, poor nutrition, lack of exercise, certain medical conditions, or age-related changes.

- **Common Symptoms:** Hormonal imbalances may manifest in a range of symptoms, including fatigue, mood swings, weight gain or loss, irregular menstrual cycles, low libido, hair loss, and sleep disturbances.

- **Health Implications:** Hormonal imbalances can contribute to the development of conditions such as polycystic ovary syndrome (PCOS), hypothyroidism, hyperthyroidism, diabetes, and infertility.

3. Impact on Health: The hormonal balance theory suggests that imbalances in hormones can have far-reaching effects on overall health and well-being.

- **Weight Management:** Hormones play a significant role in regulating metabolism and controlling appetite. Hormonal imbalances can disrupt these processes, leading to weight gain or difficulty losing weight.

- **Mood and Mental Health:** Hormonal fluctuations, particularly in estrogen and progesterone, can influence mood and contribute to conditions like premenstrual syndrome (PMS) and postpartum depression.

- **Energy Levels:** Hormonal imbalances, especially in thyroid hormones and cortisol, can impact energy levels. Low thyroid function (hypothyroidism) may result in fatigue and sluggishness, while excessive cortisol levels (as seen in chronic stress) can lead to a state of constant fatigue.

4. Management and Treatment: Addressing hormonal imbalances often involves a multifaceted approach.

- **Lifestyle Modifications:** Adopting a healthy lifestyle that includes regular exercise, a balanced diet, stress management techniques, and adequate sleep can support hormonal balance.

- **Hormone Replacement Therapy:** In some cases, hormone replacement therapy may be recommended to restore hormonal balance. This approach is commonly used in conditions like menopause or hypothyroidism.

- **Targeted Medications:** Certain medications may be prescribed to manage specific hormonal conditions. For example, birth control pills can regulate menstrual cycles and manage hormonal acne.

The Zone Ratio

The Zone Ratio is a popular dietary approach developed by Dr. Barry Sears in the 1990s. It focuses on achieving a specific macronutrient balance in order to optimize hormonal response, control inflammation, and promote overall health. The Zone Ratio is often referred to as the "40-30-30" ratio, which represents the percentage of calories that should come from carbohydrates, protein, and fat, respectively. Let's dive deeper into this concept and explore its principles and benefits.

Principles Of The Zone Ratio

The Zone Ratio is based on the principle that the balance of macronutrients in a meal or diet can impact the body's hormonal response, particularly the production of insulin, glucagon, and eicosanoids. By carefully controlling these hormonal responses, the Zone Ratio aims to achieve several health benefits, including improved energy levels, better weight management, reduced inflammation, and enhanced mental focus.

Understanding The Ideal Macronutrient Balance

The Zone Ratio recommends a balance of 40% carbohydrates, 30% protein, and 30% fat in each meal. This macronutrient distribution is believed to help stabilize blood sugar levels, control hunger, and support the body's metabolic processes. Here's a breakdown of each macronutrient and its role in the body:

1. **Carbohydrates**: Carbs are the body's primary source of energy. They provide fuel for the brain, muscles, and other organs. The Zone Ratio suggests focusing on low-glycemic carbohydrates, such as fruits, vegetables, whole grains, and legumes, which have a slower impact on blood sugar levels and promote sustained energy release.

2. **Protein**: Protein is essential for building and repairing tissues, supporting immune function, and regulating various physiological processes. It also helps to increase satiety and preserve lean muscle mass. The Zone Ratio recommends lean protein sources like poultry, fish, eggs, and plant-based proteins such as beans and tofu.

3. **Fat**: Dietary fat is crucial for hormone production, brain function, and nutrient absorption. The Zone Ratio emphasizes healthy fats, including monounsaturated fats found in olive oil, avocados, and nuts, as well as omega-3 fatty acids from fatty fish like salmon and chia seeds.

Exploring The Recommended 40-30-30 Ratio

The Zone Ratio suggests that by consuming a balanced meal with the recommended 40% carbohydrates, 30% protein, and 30% fat, individuals can regulate their insulin levels and maintain a steady blood sugar response. This is thought to prevent spikes and crashes in energy levels, reduce inflammation, and promote satiety.

1. **Carbohydrates in the Zone Ratio**: The 40% carbohydrate portion focuses on choosing complex carbs that are rich in fiber and have a low glycemic index. These include vegetables, fruits, whole grains, and legumes. By selecting carbohydrates with a lower impact on blood sugar levels, the Zone Ratio aims to avoid insulin spikes and support more stable energy throughout the day.

2. **Protein in the Zone Ratio**: The 30% protein portion in the Zone Ratio ensures an adequate intake to support muscle maintenance and repair, as well as various metabolic functions. High-quality protein sources like lean meats, fish, poultry, eggs, and plant-based proteins are recommended. Adequate protein intake is important for appetite control and promoting satiety.

3. **Fat in the Zone Ratio**: The 30% fat portion emphasizes the consumption of healthy fats, particularly those rich in monounsaturated fats and omega-3 fatty acids. These fats are believed to have anti-inflammatory properties and support overall health. Sources of healthy fats include olive oil, avocados, nuts, seeds, and fatty fish.

By adhering to the recommended 40-30-30 ratio of carbohydrates, protein, and fat, individuals following the Zone Ratio aim to create a hormonal balance that promotes optimal health and well-being. Here are some key points to consider when implementing the Zone Ratio:

1. Meal Planning: Planning meals with the Zone Ratio in mind involves selecting a variety of foods that fit within the recommended macronutrient percentages. This may require portion control and paying attention to the nutritional composition of different ingredients. It is essential to include a balance of carbohydrates, proteins, and fats in each meal.

2. Balancing Blood Sugar: The Zone Ratio emphasizes the importance of maintaining stable blood sugar levels throughout the day. By including complex carbohydrates, lean proteins, and healthy fats in meals, the aim is to avoid rapid spikes and drops in blood sugar, which can lead to energy crashes and cravings.

3. Satiety and Weight Management: The Zone Ratio aims to promote satiety and support weight management by including an adequate amount of protein and healthy fats in each meal. Protein is known to increase feelings of fullness and can help prevent overeating. Healthy fats contribute to satiety and can help regulate appetite.

4. Individualization: While the Zone Ratio provides general guidelines, it's important to recognize that individual needs may vary. Factors such as age, gender, activity level, and overall health should be considered when determining the appropriate macronutrient balance for each person. Consulting with a registered dietitian or healthcare professional can provide personalized guidance.

5. Flexibility: The Zone Ratio encourages flexibility and does not promote strict calorie counting or elimination of entire food groups. It allows for customization based on personal preferences and dietary restrictions, as long as the overall macronutrient balance is maintained. This approach makes it sustainable for long-term adherence.

6. Exercise and Lifestyle: The Zone Ratio can be complemented by regular physical activity and a healthy lifestyle. Engaging in regular exercise, managing stress levels, staying adequately hydrated, and getting sufficient sleep are all important factors that contribute to overall well-being and the success of any dietary approach.

It's worth noting that while the Zone Ratio has gained popularity and has been endorsed by some individuals, it is not without its critics. Some experts argue that the macronutrient distribution may not be suitable for everyone and that individual responses to different ratios may vary. As with any dietary approach, it's essential to listen to your body, monitor your health, and make adjustments as necessary.

CHAPTER TWO

Getting Started with The Zone

Assessing Your Current State

Assessing your current state is an important step in any journey towards health and wellness. It allows you to gain a clear understanding of where you currently stand in terms of your overall well-being, fitness level, and lifestyle choices. By taking the time to assess your current state, you can identify areas that may need improvement and set realistic goals for yourself. Let's explore some key aspects to consider when assessing your current state.

Physical Fitness: One aspect of assessing your current state is evaluating your physical fitness. This includes considering your cardiovascular endurance, muscular strength and endurance, flexibility, and body composition. Take note of your ability to perform different physical activities, such as running, lifting weights, or completing a yoga routine. Assessing your physical fitness can help you gauge your overall health and identify areas for improvement.

Mental and Emotional Well-being: It's also important to assess your mental and emotional well-being. Consider your stress levels, mood, and overall outlook on life. Take note of any signs of anxiety or depression that you may be experiencing. This evaluation can help you understand the impact of your mental and emotional state on your overall well-being and identify any areas that require attention or support.

Lifestyle Habits: Evaluating your lifestyle habits is crucial when assessing your current state. Consider your sleep patterns, hydration levels, and stress management techniques. Assess your habits related to smoking, alcohol consumption, and drug use, if applicable. Additionally, evaluate your work-life balance, relationships, and social interactions. Understanding your lifestyle habits can help you identify areas that may be negatively impacting your well-being and make necessary changes.

Medical History and Current Health Conditions: Another important aspect of assessing your current state is reviewing your medical history and any existing health conditions. Consider any chronic illnesses, injuries, or surgeries you have had in the past. Assess your current medication use and any symptoms or issues you may be facing. This evaluation can provide valuable insights into how your health conditions may be affecting your overall well-being and guide you in seeking appropriate medical support if necessary.

Nutritional Intake: Evaluating your nutritional intake is a crucial part of assessing your current state. Take a closer look at your dietary choices and habits. Consider the types of food you consume, portion sizes, and meal patterns. Assess your intake of essential nutrients, such as vitamins, minerals, and macronutrients (carbohydrates, proteins, and fats). This assessment can help you determine if your current eating habits are supporting your health goals or if adjustments are needed.

In summary, assessing your current state involves evaluating various aspects of your physical and mental well-being, lifestyle habits, medical history, and nutritional intake. By taking the time to assess these areas, you can gain a comprehensive understanding of your current state of health and make informed decisions to improve your overall well-being. Remember that this assessment is not meant to be judgmental but rather a tool to empower you on your journey towards a healthier and happier life.

Determining Your Body Fat Percentage

Determining your body fat percentage is a valuable tool in assessing your body composition and overall health. Body fat percentage refers to the proportion of fat in your body compared to your total body weight. While some amount of body fat is essential for normal bodily functions, excess body fat can increase the risk of various health conditions. Let's explore different methods for determining your body fat percentage.

Calipers: One common method used to determine body fat percentage is skinfold calipers. This technique involves using calipers to measure the thickness of skinfolds at specific body sites, such as the triceps, abdomen, and thighs. These measurements are then used in an equation to estimate body fat percentage. While calipers are relatively inexpensive and easy to use, they do require some skillS.

Bioelectrical Impedance Analysis (BIA): Bioelectrical Impedance Analysis is another method commonly used to estimate body fat percentage. BIA works by sending a low-level electrical current through the body and measuring the resistance encountered by the current. This resistance is then used to calculate body fat percentage. BIA devices are available for home use and are relatively simple to operate. However, it's important to note that factors such as hydration levels and body temperature can affect the accuracy of BIA measurements.

Dual-Energy X-ray Absorptiometry (DXA): DXA is considered one of the most accurate methods for determining body fat percentage. It uses a low-dose X-ray to measure the amount of lean tissue, fat tissue, and bone in the body. DXA scans provide detailed information about body composition and can differentiate between visceral fat (fat stored around organs) and subcutaneous fat (fat stored beneath the skin). DXA scans are usually performed in specialized clinics or hospitals and are more expensive than other methods.

Air Displacement Plethysmography (ADP): ADP, commonly known as the Bod Pod, is a method that measures body composition by calculating the amount of air displaced when a person enters a sealed chamber. By comparing the volume of air displaced with the person's body weight, body fat percentage can be estimated. ADP is a safe and non-invasive method, but it may not be as accurate as DXA for certain populations, such as athletes or individuals with significant muscle mass.

Hydrostatic Weighing: Hydrostatic weighing, also known as underwater weighing, involves submerging the body in water and measuring the displacement of water to estimate body volume. This method relies on the principle that fat is less dense than muscle and bone. Hydrostatic weighing requires specialized equipment and is typically performed in research or clinical settings. It is considered highly accurate but may not be as accessible or convenient as other methods.

It's important to note that each method for determining body fat percentage has its own strengths and limitations. The accuracy of these methods can be influenced by factors such as hydration levels, age, gender, and body composition. Furthermore, the interpretation of body fat percentage should be done in conjunction with other health indicators and individual goals.

Regardless of the method you choose, it's essential to remember that body fat percentage is just one component of overall health and should be considered in conjunction with other factors such as fitness level, muscle mass, and lifestyle habits. Consulting with a healthcare professional or a certified fitness expert can provide valuable guidance in interpreting your body fat percentage and developing a comprehensive plan to improve your overall health.

Evaluating Your Current Eating Habits And Energy Levels

Evaluating your current eating habits and energy levels is essential for understanding how your diet may be affecting your overall well-being. The food you consume plays a significant role in providing the necessary nutrients for energy, supporting bodily functions, and maintaining good health. Let's explore some key points to consider when evaluating your eating habits and energy levels.

Food Choices and Nutrient Balance: Start by assessing the types of foods you regularly consume. Are you eating a variety of whole, nutrient-dense foods such as fruits, vegetables, whole grains, lean proteins, and healthy fats? Or do your choices lean more towards processed and high-calorie foods? Evaluating your food choices can help you identify areas for improvement and make adjustments to ensure you're getting a balance of essential nutrients.

Meal Patterns and Portion Control: Consider your meal patterns and portion sizes. Are you eating three balanced meals a day, or do you tend to skip meals or rely heavily on snacks? Assessing your meal patterns can help you identify if you're getting consistent energy throughout the day. Additionally, pay attention to portion sizes to ensure you're not overeating or undereating. Finding the right balance for your individual needs is crucial for maintaining stable energy levels.

Food Quality and Macronutrient Balance: Evaluate the quality of the macronutrients in your diet - carbohydrates, proteins, and fats. Are you getting a good balance of these macronutrients? Carbohydrates provide energy, proteins support muscle growth and repair, and fats are essential for various bodily functions. Assessing the macronutrient balance in your diet can help ensure you're meeting your body's energy needs and supporting optimal health.

Hydration: Assess your hydration levels. Are you drinking enough water throughout the day? Water is essential for maintaining proper bodily functions, including digestion and energy production. Evaluate your daily water intake and make adjustments if necessary to stay adequately hydrated.

Eating Mindfully: Consider how you approach meals and snacks. Do you eat mindfully, paying attention to hunger and fullness cues? Or do you often eat out of boredom, stress, or other emotional triggers? Mindful eating involves being present and aware of your body's signals and making conscious choices about what and how much you eat. Evaluating your eating behaviors can help you identify areas where you may need to make changes to promote a healthier relationship with food.

Energy Levels: Reflect on your overall energy levels throughout the day. Do you feel consistently energized, or do you experience frequent fluctuations in energy? Evaluating your energy levels can provide insights into how your eating habits may be influencing your daily vitality. Consider if you're getting enough calories to support your activity level and if the distribution of macronutrients in your meals is helping sustain steady energy levels.

Emotional and Psychological Factors: Lastly, assess any emotional or psychological factors that may be influencing your eating habits and energy levels. Stress, boredom, or emotional eating can lead to unhealthy food choices and energy imbalances. Recognizing these factors can help you develop strategies to manage them and make more mindful choices about your nutrition.

Setting Goals

Setting goals is a crucial step in personal development and achieving success in various aspects of life. Whether it's related to career, relationships, health, or personal growth, goals provide direction and motivation. By defining clear objectives, you can effectively plan your actions, track your progress, and stay focused on the desired outcome. In this article, we will explore the importance of setting goals, discuss how to define weight loss and energy improvement goals, and emphasize the significance of establishing realistic targets for success.

Importance Of Setting Goals

Setting goals provides several benefits that contribute to personal growth and success. Here are a few key reasons why setting goals is essential:

1. **Clarity**: Goals provide clarity by defining the desired outcome. They give you a clear picture of what you want to achieve and help you focus your efforts and resources accordingly.

2. **Motivation**: Goals act as powerful motivators. They provide a sense of purpose and drive, fueling your determination and perseverance. Having a specific target in mind keeps you motivated during challenging times.

3. **Direction**: Goals serve as a roadmap, guiding your

actions and decisions. They help you prioritize tasks, allocate resources effectively, and avoid distractions that might hinder your progress.

4. **Measurability**: Setting goals allows you to measure your progress objectively. By breaking down your larger objectives into smaller, measurable milestones, you can track your advancement and celebrate your achievements along the way.

5. **Accountability**: Goals create a sense of accountability. When you set goals, you commit to taking specific actions and achieving certain outcomes. This commitment holds you responsible for your own success.

Defining Weight Loss And Energy Improvement Goals

When it comes to health and well-being, setting goals for weight loss and energy improvement is common. Defining these goals requires careful consideration and a realistic approach. Here are some steps to help you define your weight loss and energy improvement goals effectively:

1. **Assess your current state**: Begin by assessing your current weight and energy levels. Consider any health issues or lifestyle factors that might be impacting your weight and energy. Understanding your starting point will help you set appropriate and realistic goals.

2. **Identify desired outcomes**: Determine what you

want to achieve regarding weight loss and energy improvement. Be specific about the results you desire, such as losing a certain amount of weight or feeling more energized throughout the day.

3. **Break it down**: Once you have identified your desired outcomes, break them down into smaller, manageable goals. This allows you to focus on one step at a time, making your overall objective less overwhelming.

4. **Set SMART goals**: Make sure your goals are SMART: Specific, Measurable, Achievable, Relevant, and Time-bound. For example, instead of saying, "I want to lose weight," a SMART goal would be, "I will lose 10 pounds in the next three months by following a balanced diet and exercising three times a week."

5. **Consider lifestyle changes**: To support your weight loss and energy improvement goals, consider making sustainable lifestyle changes. This might include adopting a nutritious diet, incorporating regular exercise, getting enough sleep, and managing stress effectively.

Establishing Realistic Targets For Success

While setting ambitious goals can be motivating, it's crucial to establish realistic targets for success. Unrealistic goals can lead to disappointment, frustration, and a higher likelihood of giving up. Here are some guidelines for setting realistic targets:

1. **Be aware of your limitations**: Consider your current circumstances, commitments, and resources. Set goals that align with your capabilities and take into account any constraints you might have, such as time, finances, or physical abilities.

2. **Focus on gradual progress**: Instead of aiming for rapid and drastic changes, focus on gradual progress. Setting small, gradual and achievable targets allows for sustainable progress and reduces the risk of burnout or setbacks. For example, aiming to lose 1-2 pounds per week is a more realistic and healthy target than trying to lose 10 pounds in a week.

3. **Consider your personal circumstances**: Everyone's journey is unique, and what works for one person may not work for another. Take into account your age, body composition, metabolism, and any underlying health conditions when setting your targets. Consulting with a healthcare professional or a registered dietitian can provide valuable guidance tailored to your specific needs.

4. **Track your progress**: Regularly monitor and track your progress towards your goals. This allows you to assess whether you're on track or need to make adjustments. Keep a journal, use tracking apps, or take measurements to objectively measure your progress.

5. **Celebrate milestones**: Acknowledge and celebrate your achievements along the way. Recognizing your progress and small victories can boost your motivation and reinforce positive habits. Reward

yourself with non-food rewards, such as a new workout outfit or a spa day, to stay motivated and focused.

6. **Be flexible and adaptable**: It's important to be flexible and adapt your goals as needed. Life can throw unexpected challenges, and it's okay to modify your targets if necessary. Listen to your body and make adjustments if you're experiencing excessive fatigue or any health concerns.

7. **Stay positive and maintain a growth mindset**: Maintaining a positive mindset is crucial for long-term success. Embrace setbacks as learning opportunities and approach challenges with a growth mindset. Focus on the progress you've made and the habits you've developed rather than solely on the end result.

Creating A Zone-Friendly Pantry

When it comes to following the Zone diet, creating a pantry that is conducive to this eating plan is essential. The Zone diet, developed by Dr. Barry Sears, focuses on balancing macronutrients to optimize hormone levels and promote weight loss. The goal is to maintain a steady balance of protein, carbohydrates, and fats in each meal to stabilize blood sugar levels and control hunger. To create a Zone-friendly pantry, here are a few key steps to consider:

1. **Clear out non-Zone foods**: Begin by removing any foods from your pantry that are not approved

for the Zone diet. This includes processed foods, sugary snacks, refined grains, and unhealthy fats. By eliminating these items, you eliminate the temptation to stray from the Zone guidelines.

2. **Stock up on fresh produce**: Fresh fruits and vegetables should form the foundation of your Zone-friendly pantry. These nutrient-dense foods provide essential vitamins, minerals, and fiber while being low in calories. Aim to include a variety of colorful options to ensure a wide range of nutrients.

3. **Choose lean proteins**: The Zone diet emphasizes the consumption of lean proteins, such as chicken, turkey, fish, tofu, and legumes. These protein sources are low in saturated fats and rich in essential amino acids. Consider stocking up on canned beans and legumes for quick and easy meal options.

4. **Include healthy fats**: While the Zone diet restricts the consumption of unhealthy fats, it encourages the intake of healthy fats. Opt for sources like avocados, nuts, seeds, olive oil, and fatty fish like salmon. These fats are important for brain health, hormone production, and overall well-being.

5. **Select complex carbohydrates**: In the Zone diet, carbohydrates should come from sources that have a low glycemic index to prevent spikes in blood sugar levels. Focus on whole grains, such as brown rice, quinoa, oats, and whole wheat bread. These provide sustained energy and a steady release of glucose into the bloodstream.

6. **Minimize processed foods**: Processed foods are often high in added sugars, unhealthy fats, and artificial additives. These can disrupt the hormonal balance that the Zone diet aims to achieve. Instead, choose whole, unprocessed foods as much as possible to ensure optimal nutrition.

7. **Read labels**: When stocking your Zone-friendly pantry, be sure to read the labels of packaged foods. Look for items with minimal ingredients, no added sugars, and no trans fats. Check the macronutrient breakdown to ensure it aligns with the Zone diet's guidelines.

By following these steps, you can create a pantry that is aligned with the Zone diet principles. Remember to regularly assess and restock your pantry to ensure you have a variety of Zone-approved options readily available.

Identifying Zone-Approved Foods

To successfully follow the Zone diet, it is crucial to be able to identify foods that are approved for the diet. The Zone diet focuses on balancing macronutrients in a specific ratio to promote hormonal balance and control hunger. Here are some guidelines for identifying Zone-approved foods:

1. **Proteins**: Zone-approved proteins should be low in fat and provide essential amino acids. Lean sources of protein include chicken breast, turkey breast, fish (such as salmon and tuna), tofu, egg

whites, and low-fat dairy products (like cottage cheese and Greek yogurt). Avoid fatty cuts of meat and processed meats, as they may contain unhealthy fats and additives.

2. **Carbohydrates** (continued): As mentioned earlier, non-starchy vegetables and whole grains are excellent choices for Zone-approved carbohydrates. Additionally, include fruits like berries, apples, and citrus fruits in moderation, as they provide essential vitamins, minerals, and fiber. It's important to note that the Zone diet recommends controlling the portion sizes of carbohydrates to maintain the desired macronutrient balance.

3. **Fats**: The Zone diet emphasizes the consumption of healthy fats while limiting unhealthy fats. Opt for monounsaturated fats found in avocados, olive oil, nuts (such as almonds and walnuts), and seeds (like flaxseeds and chia seeds). Omega-3 fatty acids, found in fatty fish like salmon and trout, are also beneficial for their anti-inflammatory properties. Limit the intake of saturated fats found in high-fat dairy products and fatty cuts of meat.

4. **Snacks**: When it comes to Zone-approved snacks, focus on incorporating a combination of protein, carbohydrates, and fats. For example, you can have a handful of almonds (protein and healthy fats) with a piece of fruit (carbohydrates). Greek yogurt with berries or raw vegetables with hummus are other options that provide a balanced nutrient profile. Avoid sugary snacks

and processed foods that can disrupt the hormonal balance the Zone diet aims to achieve.

5. **Beverages**: While water is the best choice for hydration, you can also include other Zone-friendly beverages. Herbal teas, unsweetened green tea, and black coffee without added sugars or cream are acceptable. Avoid sugary drinks, sodas, and fruit juices, as they can cause blood sugar imbalances.

6. **Condiments and seasonings**: Pay attention to the condiments and seasonings you use to flavor your meals. Choose options that are low in added sugars and unhealthy fats. Herbs, spices, vinegar, mustard, and small amounts of low-sodium soy sauce can enhance the taste of your dishes without compromising the Zone-approved guidelines.

Remember that portion control and balance are key principles of the Zone diet. It's important to consult with a healthcare professional or registered dietitian before starting any new diet plan, as individual needs may vary.

Stocking Up On Essential Ingredients

When following a specific diet plan like the Zone diet, having a well-stocked pantry with essential ingredients is crucial. It ensures that you have the necessary items on hand to prepare balanced meals and stick to the guidelines of the diet. Here are some essential ingredients to stock up on for the Zone diet:

1. **Proteins**: Lean proteins should be a staple in your pantry. Chicken breast, turkey breast, fish (such as salmon and tuna), lean cuts of beef or pork, tofu, tempeh, legumes (like lentils and beans), and low-fat dairy products (such as Greek yogurt and cottage cheese) are excellent options. Choose sources that are low in saturated fat and provide essential amino acids.

2. **Fruits and vegetables**: Fresh or frozen fruits and vegetables are essential for a Zone-friendly pantry. Aim for a variety of non-starchy vegetables, such as broccoli, spinach, kale, bell peppers, cucumbers, and cauliflower. Include fruits like berries, apples, oranges, and grapefruits. Having frozen options available can be convenient when fresh produce is not readily available.

3. **Whole grains and legumes**: Whole grains like brown rice, quinoa, oats, and whole wheat products should be included in moderation. These provide a good source of fiber and complex carbohydrates. Legumes, such as lentils, chickpeas, and black beans, are also beneficial for their protein and fiber content. Opt for whole grain options like quinoa, brown rice, whole wheat bread, and whole wheat pasta. These provide sustained energy and fiber. Legumes, such as lentils, chickpeas, and black beans, are great sources of plant-based protein and fiber.

3. **Healthy fats**: Include a variety of healthy fats in your pantry. Olive oil, avocado oil, nuts (such

as almonds, walnuts, and pistachios), seeds (like flaxseeds, chia seeds, and hemp seeds), and nut butter (without added sugars) are excellent choices. These fats help support brain health, hormone production, and overall well-being.

4. **Low-fat dairy products**: If you consume dairy, opt for low-fat options like Greek yogurt, cottage cheese, and skim milk. These provide protein and calcium without excess saturated fat. Be mindful of added sugars in flavored varieties, and choose plain options that you can flavor yourself with fruits or a small amount of honey.

5. **Herbs, spices, and condiments**: Stock your pantry with a variety of herbs and spices to add flavor to your meals without relying on excessive salt or sauces. Options like basil, oregano, garlic powder, paprika, cumin, and turmeric can enhance the taste of your dishes. Condiments like mustard, hot sauce (without added sugars), vinegar, and low-sodium soy sauce are also handy for adding flavor.

6. **Nuts and seeds**: Keep a selection of nuts and seeds on hand for snacking or adding to meals. Almonds, walnuts, cashews, chia seeds, flaxseeds, and sunflower seeds are nutritious options that provide healthy fats, protein, and fiber. Remember to consume them in moderation, as they are calorie-dense.

7. **Canned goods**: Canned beans, such as black beans, kidney beans, and chickpeas, are convenient pantry staples. They are a good source of protein and fiber and can be used in a variety of dishes

like salads, soups, and stews. Opt for low-sodium versions and rinse them before using to reduce the sodium content.

8. **Protein powders**: While not necessary, having a high-quality protein powder can be beneficial for meeting your protein needs, especially for those who have higher protein requirements or find it challenging to get enough protein from whole foods alone. Look for options that are low in added sugars and artificial ingredients.

9. **Freezer essentials**: Apart from frozen fruits and vegetables, consider stocking your freezer with lean meats, poultry, and fish. These can be easily thawed and used for quick and healthy meals. Additionally, frozen shrimp, edamame, and pre-portioned meals can be convenient options.

CHAPTER THREE

The Zone Meal Planning

The Basics Of Zone Meals

The Zone Diet, developed by Dr. Barry Sears, is a popular eating plan that emphasizes balancing macronutrients to achieve optimal health and weight management. The concept behind Zone meals is to consume a specific ratio of carbohydrates, proteins, and fats at every meal to keep blood sugar levels stable and promote a balanced metabolism. By structuring your meals in this way, you can potentially control hunger, improve energy levels, and enhance overall well-being.

1. The 40-30-30 Ratio: One of the key principles of Zone meals is maintaining a specific macronutrient ratio of 40% carbohydrates, 30% protein, and 30% fat. This balance is believed to optimize hormone levels and stabilize blood sugar, which can lead to increased fat loss and improved body composition. By adhering to this ratio, you can ensure that your meals are well-rounded and provide the necessary nutrients for your body's needs.

2. Zone Blocks: To make meal planning easier, the Zone Diet employs a system called Zone blocks. Each macronutrient is assigned a specific block value, which represents a set amount of that particular nutrient. For example, one block of protein is equivalent to 7 grams, one block of carbohydrates is equal to 9 grams, and one block of fat is around 1.5 grams. By using these block measurements, you can easily create balanced meals that adhere to the 40-30-30 ratio.

3. Portion Control: Zone meals also emphasize portion control to maintain the appropriate balance of macronutrients. The number of blocks you should consume per meal depends on various factors such as your body weight, activity level, and goals. Typically, women might start with three blocks per meal, while men might begin with four blocks. These portions can be adjusted based on individual needs and progress.

4. Meal Frequency: Another aspect of the Zone Diet is spreading out meals and snacks throughout the day. This eating pattern involves having three meals and two snacks, each containing the appropriate number of blocks. By eating every few hours, you can help stabilize blood sugar levels and prevent energy crashes. This approach also prevents overeating and ensures a steady supply of nutrients for your body.

5. Food Choices: While the Zone Diet doesn't restrict any particular food groups, it encourages selecting nutrient-dense and low-glycemic index foods. These include lean proteins, fruits, vegetables, whole grains, and healthy fats. The focus is on consuming high-quality carbohydrates, such as colorful vegetables and low-sugar fruits, which are slower to digest and provide sustained energy.

6. Benefits and Considerations: Proponents of the Zone Diet claim that following Zone meals can lead to weight loss, improved athletic performance, reduced inflammation, and better overall health. However, it's important to note that individual responses may vary, and the diet may not be suitable for everyone. Some people may find it challenging to adhere to the strict macronutrient ratios or may require additional customization based on their specific needs or dietary restrictions.

In conclusion, Zone meals are centered around balancing macronutrients in a specific ratio to optimize health and weight management. By using Zone blocks and portion control, you can create well-rounded meals that provide a steady supply of nutrients throughout the day. However, it's essential to consult with a healthcare professional or registered dietitian before starting any new dietary regimen to ensure it aligns with your individual needs and goals.

Understanding Zone Blocks And Portion Sizes

In the Zone Diet, Zone blocks are a fundamental aspect used to guide portion sizes and ensure a balanced distribution of macronutrients in meals. By understanding how Zone blocks work, you can effectively plan and create meals that align with the Zone Diet principles. Here's a closer look at

Zone blocks and how they help in portion control:

1. What are Zone Blocks? Zone blocks are a measurement system used in the Zone Diet to quantify the amounts of macronutrients in different foods. Each macronutrient category (protein, carbohydrates, and fats) is assigned a specific block value. These values are standardized to make it easier for individuals to create balanced meals based on their individual needs and goals.

2. Protein Zone Blocks: Protein is an essential macronutrient for muscle repair and growth. In the Zone Diet, one protein block is equal to 7 grams of protein. Common sources of protein that can be used to measure a block include chicken breast, lean beef, fish, tofu, or eggs. For example, if a meal calls for three protein blocks, you would aim to consume 21 grams of protein from your chosen protein sources.

3. Carbohydrate Zone Blocks: Carbohydrates are the body's primary source of energy. In the Zone Diet, one carbohydrate block is equivalent to 9 grams of carbohydrates. Foods like fruits, vegetables, whole grains, and legumes can be used to measure a carbohydrate block. For instance, if a meal requires two carbohydrate blocks, you would aim to consume 18 grams of carbohydrates from these sources.

4. Fat Zone Blocks: Fats play various roles in the body, including providing energy, supporting hormone production, and aiding in nutrient absorption. In the Zone

Diet, one fat block is approximately 1.5 grams of fat. Healthy fat sources such as nuts, seeds, avocado, olive oil, and fatty fish can be used to measure a fat block. For example, if a meal calls for four fat blocks, you would aim to consume around 6 grams of fat from these sources.

5. Customization and Adjustments: The number of Zone blocks you should consume per meal depends on factors like your gender, weight, activity level, and goals. For example, women typically start with three blocks of protein, carbohydrates, and fats per meal, while men might begin with four blocks. However, these values can be adjusted based on individual needs and progress.

6. Creating Zone Meals: To create Zone meals, you need to combine the appropriate number of Zone blocks from each macronutrient category. For example, a meal might consist of three protein blocks, two carbohydrate blocks, and four fat blocks, following the 40-30-30 ratio. This ensures a balanced distribution of macronutrients, which is believed to help stabilize blood sugar levels and promote overall well-being.

7. Meal Planning and Flexibility: Meal planning is crucial for success on the Zone Diet. By prepping and portioning your meals ahead of time, you can ensure that you're consuming the right number of Zone blocks per meal. It's important to note that the Zone Diet allows for flexibility in food choices, as long as you adhere to the appropriate macronutrient ratios. This means you can customize your meals based on personal preferences and dietary restrictions.

8. Consulting a Professional: While understanding Zone blocks and portion sizes is essential for following the Zone Diet, it's always recommended to consult with a healthcare professional or registered dietitian. They can help assess your specific needs, guide you in creating personalized Zone meals, and address any concerns or questions you may have.

Planning Meals With Balanced Macronutrients

Planning meals with balanced macronutrients is a key component of the Zone Diet. By focusing on the appropriate ratio of carbohydrates, proteins, and fats, you can optimize your nutrient intake and support overall health. Here's a closer look at how to plan meals with balanced macronutrients:

1. Determine Your Zone Block Requirements: Before planning your meals, it's essential to determine the number of Zone blocks you need per meal based on your gender, weight, activity level, and goals. As mentioned earlier, women typically start with three blocks per meal, while men start with four blocks. However, these numbers can be adjusted to suit your individual needs and progress.

2. Choose High-Quality Protein Sources: Protein is an essential macronutrient that supports muscle growth, repair, and various bodily functions. When planning your meals, opt for lean sources of protein such as chicken breast, turkey, fish, tofu, legumes, and low-fat dairy products. These options provide essential amino acids without adding excessive amounts of unhealthy fats.

3. Incorporate Colorful Vegetables and Fruits: Vegetables and fruits are excellent sources of fiber, vitamins, and minerals. Aim to include a variety of colorful options in your meals to ensure a wide range of nutrients. Choose low-glycemic index vegetables like leafy greens, broccoli, peppers, and tomatoes, as they have a minimal impact on blood sugar levels. Similarly, opt for lower-sugar fruits such as berries, apples, and citrus fruits.

4. Include Complex Carbohydrates: Complex carbohydrates are digested more slowly, providing a steady release of energy and helping to keep blood sugar levels stable. Examples of complex carbohydrates include whole grains like brown rice, quinoa, oats, and whole wheat products. These should be portioned according to your Zone block requirements, ensuring you're getting an adequate amount of carbohydrates while maintaining the 40% ratio.

5. Incorporate Healthy Fats: While fats should be consumed in moderation, it's important to include healthy sources of fats in your meals. These include avocados, nuts, seeds, olive oil, and fatty fish like salmon and tuna. These fats provide essential fatty acids and help promote satiety. Remember to measure your fat portions according to the Zone block requirements to maintain the 30% fat ratio.

6. Plan Balanced Meals with Zone Blocks: Once you have determined your Zone block requirements and chosen appropriate protein, carbohydrate, and fat sources, you can start planning your meals. Aim to include the specified number of Zone blocks for each macronutrient in every meal, ensuring that you maintain the 40-30-30 ratio. For example, if you are allotted three blocks per meal, you might have three protein blocks, three carbohydrate blocks, and three fat blocks.

7. Snack Options: In addition to your main meals, you can also plan Zone-approved snacks to keep you satisfied between meals. Opt for protein-rich options like Greek yogurt, cottage cheese, hard-boiled eggs, or protein bars that are within your allotted Zone block requirements.

8. Hydration and Beverages: While the Zone Diet primarily focuses on macronutrients, it's important to stay hydrated throughout the day. Water should be your primary beverage choice. However, you can also include calorie-free beverages such as herbal tea, black coffee, or unsweetened flavored water. Avoid sugary drinks and limit your intake of alcohol.

9. Monitor and Adjust as Needed: Regularly monitor your progress and make adjustments to your meal planning as needed. Pay attention to how your body responds to different meals and adjust your portion sizes or food choices accordingly. Keep track of your energy levels, hunger, and overall well-being to fine-tune your meals and ensure they align with your goals.

10. Seek Professional Guidance: While planning meals with balanced macronutrients can be done independently, it is beneficial to consult with a registered dietitian or nutritionist. They can provide personalized guidance based on your unique needs, help you create a meal plan that suits your lifestyle, and offer support throughout your journey.

11. Considerations and Adaptations: It's important to note that the Zone Diet may not be suitable for everyone. Some individuals, such as athletes with higher energy requirements or those with specific dietary restrictions, may need to make adaptations to the standard Zone block recommendations. Consulting a healthcare professional or registered dietitian can help you tailor the Zone Diet to fit your specific needs.

12. Variety and Mindful Eating: While planning balanced meals, aim for variety to ensure you receive a wide range of nutrients. Incorporate different food groups, experiment with flavors and cooking methods, and try new recipes to keep your meals interesting and enjoyable. Additionally, practicing mindful eating can help you appreciate the flavors and textures of your food, enhance digestion, and promote better overall satisfaction.

13. Long-Term Sustainability: When planning meals with balanced macronutrients, it's essential to consider the long-term sustainability of your approach. The Zone Diet encourages a balanced and flexible approach to eating, which can be maintained over the long term. Focus on building healthy habits, making gradual changes, and finding a meal plan that fits your lifestyle and preferences.

Building Zone-Friendly Meals

When it comes to optimizing our daily nutrition, building zone-friendly meals is a smart approach. The concept of "zone" refers to achieving a balanced macronutrient ratio in our diet, specifically focusing on the proportions of protein, carbohydrates, and fats. By creating meals that align with this zone framework, we can promote stable blood sugar levels, sustained energy, and overall well-being. Let's explore some strategies for building zone-friendly meals.

1. Prioritize Protein

Protein is an essential macronutrient that plays a crucial role in muscle growth, repair, and various metabolic processes. When selecting protein sources, aim for lean options that provide high-quality protein without excessive saturated fats. Some excellent choices include skinless poultry, fish, seafood, lean cuts of beef or pork, eggs, and plant-based sources like legumes, tofu, tempeh, and seitan. These options offer a good balance of amino acids while minimizing unhealthy fats.

2. Opt for Quality Carbohydrates

Carbohydrates are a valuable energy source, but not all carbs are created equal. To make zone-friendly choices, focus on selecting complex carbohydrates that provide sustained energy and essential nutrients. Whole grains like quinoa, brown rice, oats, and whole wheat products are excellent options. Include plenty of fruits and vegetables in your meals, as they offer a wide range of vitamins, minerals, and dietary fiber. Avoid refined carbohydrates like white bread, sugary snacks, and processed foods, as they can cause rapid blood sugar spikes and subsequent crashes.

3. Mindful Fats

While fats have been vilified in the past, it's important to include healthy fats in our diet for optimal health. Opt for unsaturated fats found in sources like avocados, nuts, seeds, and olive oil. These fats can support heart health and help absorb fat-soluble vitamins. However, it's essential to moderate your fat intake, as fats are calorie-dense. Be mindful of portion sizes and avoid excessive consumption of saturated and trans fats, typically found in fried foods, fatty cuts of meat, and processed snacks.

4. Balance and Portion Control

To create zone-friendly meals, it's essential to find the right balance between protein, carbohydrates, and fats. The Zone Diet, popularized by Dr. Barry Sears, suggests a macronutrient ratio of 40% carbohydrates,

30% protein, and 30% fat for optimal performance and overall well-being. However, individual needs may vary, so it's important to listen to your body and make adjustments accordingly. Consulting a registered dietitian or nutritionist can provide personalized guidance based on your specific goals and requirements.

5. Meal Prepping and Planning

An effective way to ensure zone-friendly meals is through meal prepping and planning. Set aside dedicated time each week to prepare meals and snacks in advance. This approach allows you to have control over the ingredients and portion sizes, reducing the likelihood of making impulsive, less nutritious food choices. Plan your meals around lean protein sources, whole grains, and a variety of fruits and vegetables. Having a well-stocked pantry with nutritious staples also makes it easier to build zone-friendly meals on the go.

6. Experiment with Flavor and Variety

Building zone-friendly meals doesn't mean sacrificing taste and variety. Explore different herbs, spices, and marinades to enhance the flavor of your meals. Incorporate a wide range of vegetables to add color, texture, and nutrients to your dishes. By experimenting with different recipes and ingredients, you can keep your meals exciting and enjoyable, making it easier to stick to a balanced eating plan in the long term.

Choosing the right protein sources is crucial for building a healthy and balanced diet. Protein is essential for numerous bodily functions, including muscle growth, repair, and hormone production. When aiming to select lean protein sources, it's important to consider both animal and plant-based options. Let's explore some strategies for making wise choices when it comes to protein.

1. Lean Animal Protein Sources

Animal protein sources are rich in essential amino acids, vitamins, and minerals. However, some animal products can be high in saturated fats, so it's important to opt for leaner options. Here are some lean animal protein sources to consider:

- Poultry: Skinless chicken breast and turkey breast are excellent choices as they are low in fat and high in protein.

- Fish and Seafood: Fish like salmon, trout, tuna, and sardines are not only great sources of protein but also provide heart-healthy omega-3 fatty acids. Shrimp, scallops, and other shellfish are also low in fat and high in protein.

- Lean Cuts of Meat: When selecting red meat, opt for lean cuts such as sirloin, tenderloin, or eye of round. Trim visible fat before cooking to reduce saturated fat content.

2. Plant-Based Protein Sources

Plant-based protein sources are valuable for those following vegetarian or vegan diets, or for individuals looking to incorporate more plant-based options into their meals. Here are some plant-based protein sources to consider:

- Legumes: Beans, lentils, chickpeas, and peas are excellent sources of plant-based protein. They are also high in dietary fiber, which promotes satiety and supports digestive health.

- Tofu and Tempeh: These soy-based products are versatile and can be used in various recipes. They provide a good amount of protein along with other essential nutrients.

- Seitan: Made from wheat gluten, seitan is a high-protein option for those who are not gluten-sensitive. It has a meat-like texture and can be used as a substitute in many dishes.

3. Dairy and Dairy Alternatives

Dairy products are another source of protein, but it's important to choose low-fat or fat-free options to minimize saturated fat intake. Greek yogurt, cottage cheese, and skim milk are examples of lean dairy choices. For those who are lactose intolerant or prefer dairy alternatives, options like almond milk, soy milk, and plant-based yogurts fortified with protein can provide suitable alternatives.

4. Combining Protein Sources

To optimize protein intake, it can be beneficial to combine different protein sources in your meals. For example, pairing a grain such as quinoa or brown rice with beans or tofu creates a complete protein profile. Combining complementary plant-based proteins helps ensure you receive all the essential amino acids your body needs.

5. Watch Your Cooking Methods

While selecting lean protein sources is important, it's equally crucial to consider how you prepare them. Cooking methods can significantly impact the overall fat content of the protein. Opt for grilling, baking, steaming, or broiling instead of frying or deep-frying, as these methods require minimal added fats. If you do choose to pan-fry, use healthier cooking oils like olive oil or coconut oil sparingly.

6. Consider Sustainability and Animal Welfare

In addition to nutritional considerations, some individuals may prioritize sustainability and animal welfare when selecting protein sources. Opting for sustainably sourced seafood, ethically raised poultry, and grass-fed beef can align with these values. Additionally, incorporating more plant-based protein sources into your diet can have a positive impact on the environment.

In conclusion, selecting lean protein sources is an important aspect of building a healthy and balanced diet. By incorporating

Meal Prepping For Success

Meal prepping is a valuable practice that can help individuals save time, eat healthier, and achieve their dietary goals. Whether you're aiming to lose weight, gain muscle, or simply maintain a balanced diet, effective meal prepping can set you up for success. By planning and preparing your meals in advance, you can avoid impulsive food choices and ensure that nutritious options are readily available. Here are some key strategies to consider for meal prepping success:

1. Set Clear Goals: Before you start meal prepping, define your objectives. Determine the number of meals you want to prep, the specific dietary requirements you need to meet, and the duration for which you'll be prepping. This will help you create a realistic plan and stay focused throughout the process.

2. Plan Your Meals: Begin by selecting recipes that align with your goals and preferences. Consider incorporating a variety of proteins, grains, fruits, and vegetables to ensure a well-rounded diet. Look for recipes that can be easily scaled up or down based on the number of servings you need.

3. Make a Shopping List: Once you have your meal plan in place, create a comprehensive shopping list. Take inventory of your pantry and fridge to identify ingredients you already have and those that need to be replenished. By organizing your list based on the layout of your grocery store, you can streamline your shopping experience and reduce the risk of forgetting essential items.

4. Prepare in Batches: Efficient meal preparation often involves cooking in batches. Choose a specific day or time during the week dedicated to prepping multiple meals at once. This approach saves time and energy since you can take advantage of shared ingredients and utensils. Invest in quality food storage containers that are suitable for both refrigeration and freezing.

5. Utilize Time-Saving Techniques: Look for ways to simplify your meal prepping routine. For instance, consider using pre-cut vegetables, canned beans, or frozen fruits. Additionally, using kitchen gadgets like slow cookers, rice cookers, or pressure cookers can help expedite the cooking process.

6. Portion Control: When dividing your meals into portions, pay attention to appropriate serving sizes. Use a food scale or measuring cups to ensure accuracy. Portioning your meals in advance not only helps with maintaining portion control but also makes it easier to grab a meal and go.

7. Create a Meal Schedule: Designate specific meals for each day of the week and plan accordingly. This approach helps to ensure that you have a variety of meals and prevents boredom from eating the same thing every day. It also allows you to take into account any specific events or occasions where you may need to adjust your meal plan.

8. Label and Date Containers: To keep track of freshness and avoid confusion, label each container with the meal name and date of preparation. This practice ensures that you consume meals within their recommended storage timeframes and helps prevent food waste.

9. Rotate Your Menu: To avoid monotony, consider rotating your meal options on a weekly or bi-weekly basis. This keeps your taste buds engaged and prevents boredom from setting in. Experiment with different flavors, cuisines, and cooking methods to add variety to your meals.

10. Stay Organized: Establish a system for organizing your prepped meals in the refrigerator and freezer. Designate a specific area or shelf for easy access and visibility. This will prevent your meals from getting buried or forgotten, allowing you to efficiently grab the meal you need.

Batch Cooking And Storage Strategies

Batch cooking is a fantastic technique for meal prepping,

as it allows you to prepare larger quantities of food at once, saving you time and effort in the long run.

Batch cooking involves preparing multiple servings of a particular dish or ingredient that can be utilized in various meals throughout the week. This strategy not only reduces the time spent in the kitchen but also promotes efficient storage and ensures a variety of meals. Here are some batch cooking and storage strategies to enhance your meal prepping experience:

1. Choose Batch-Friendly Recipes: Select recipes that are suitable for batch cooking. Look for dishes that can be easily scaled up and have ingredients that can withstand refrigeration or freezing without compromising their taste and texture. Soups, stews, casseroles, and roasted vegetables are excellent options for batch cooking.

2. Cook Protein in Bulk: Prepare a large batch of proteins, such as grilled chicken, baked tofu, or roasted salmon, that can be used in multiple meals. Cook the proteins plain or season them with versatile spices to allow for different flavor profiles when incorporating them into various recipes.

3. Cook Grains and Legumes in Bulk: Grains and legumes are staples in many meals and can be cooked in bulk to save time. Prepare a large quantity of rice, quinoa, lentils, or beans and store them in separate containers. This way, you can easily add them to salads, stir-fries, or grain bowls throughout the week.

4. Utilize Sheet Pan and One-Pot Meals: Sheet pan meals and one-pot dishes are ideal for batch cooking as they allow you to cook an entire meal on a single pan or pot. Simply arrange a variety of vegetables, proteins, and seasonings on a sheet pan and roast them together. Alternatively, cook all the ingredients in a single pot for a flavorful one-pot meal.

5. Properly Portion and Package: After batch cooking, portion your meals into individual servings for easy grab-and-go convenience. Use airtight containers that are suitable for refrigeration or freezing. Ensure that each container is properly sealed to maintain freshness and prevent freezer burn.

6. Label and Date Containers: To avoid confusion, label each container with the name of the dish and the date it was prepared. This helps you keep track of the freshness of your meals and ensures that you consume them within a safe storage period. Use adhesive labels or write directly on the containers with a marker.

7. Freezing Strategies: Freezing is a valuable tool for preserving batch-cooked meals. If you don't plan to consume a particular dish within a few days, divide it into individual portions and freeze them. Make sure to cool the food completely before transferring it to the freezer. Consider using freezer-safe bags or containers for efficient storage.

8. Proper Thawing Techniques: When it's time to enjoy

your frozen batch-cooked meals, it's essential to thaw them properly to maintain their quality. Ideally, thaw frozen meals in the refrigerator overnight. Alternatively, you can use the defrost function on your microwave, following the manufacturer's instructions. Avoid thawing at room temperature to minimize the risk of bacterial growth.

9. Repurpose Leftovers: Batch-cooked meals often result in leftovers, which can be repurposed into new dishes to add variety to your meals. For example, leftover roasted vegetables can be turned into a flavorful frittata or added to a salad. Get creative and find ways to transform your leftovers into exciting new meals.

10. Rotation and Meal Planning: To prevent monotony, incorporate a rotation system into your meal planning. Have a clear plan for utilizing your batch-cooked meals throughout the week. Create a schedule that ensures you're not eating the same dishes consecutively, giving you a diverse range of meals to enjoy.

CHAPTER FOUR

Implementing The Zone Lifestyle

Overcoming Common Challenges

Facing challenges is a natural part of life, and it is important to develop strategies to overcome them. Whether you are tackling personal goals, professional aspirations, or everyday obstacles, understanding how to overcome common challenges can greatly enhance your chances of success.

1. Embrace a Growth Mindset: One of the key elements in overcoming challenges is adopting a growth mindset. This perspective acknowledges that abilities and skills can be developed through dedication and effort. By viewing challenges as opportunities for growth and learning, you can approach them with a positive attitude and a determination to find solutions.

2. Set Clear and Realistic Goals: Clearly defining your goals is essential when facing challenges. Break down larger goals into smaller, manageable tasks to avoid feeling overwhelmed. Establishing specific, measurable, attainable, relevant, and time-bound (SMART) goals helps you stay focused and track your progress along the way.

3. Seek Support: Don't hesitate to reach out for support when facing challenges. Discussing your situation with friends, family, or mentors can provide valuable insights and different perspectives. They may have faced similar challenges in the past and can offer guidance, encouragement, and assistance.

4. Develop Problem-Solving Skills: Enhancing your problem-solving skills is crucial when overcoming challenges. Break down the problem into smaller parts, analyze each component, and brainstorm potential solutions. Evaluate the pros and cons of each option and choose the one that seems most feasible. Over time, practice and experience will sharpen your problem-solving abilities.

5. Learn from Failure: Failure is an inevitable part of life, but it can be a powerful teacher. Instead of being discouraged by setbacks, use them as opportunities for growth and learning. Reflect on what went wrong, identify areas for improvement, and adjust your approach accordingly. Remember that many successful individuals have faced numerous failures before achieving their goals.

6. Practice Self-Care: Taking care of your physical and mental well-being is essential for overcoming challenges. Engage in activities that reduce stress, such as exercise, meditation, or hobbies you enjoy. Prioritize self-care to maintain your energy, focus, and resilience in the face of challenges.

7. Stay Persistent and Resilient: Challenges often require persistence and resilience to overcome. Expect obstacles along the way, and don't let setbacks discourage you. Stay committed to your goals, remain adaptable, and keep pushing forward. Remember that perseverance is key to achieving long-term success.

Dealing With Cravings And Hunger Pangs

Cravings and hunger pangs can be common obstacles when trying to maintain a healthy diet or reach specific health goals. Understanding how to manage these urges effectively can support your overall well-being and make it easier to stick to your dietary plans.

1. Identify the Triggers: Cravings can be triggered by various factors, such as emotions, social situations, or specific foods. Pay attention to what circumstances or emotions tend to trigger your cravings. By recognizing these triggers, you can develop strategies to address them proactively.

2. Distinguish Between Physical and Emotional Hunger: It is important to differentiate between physical hunger and emotional hunger. Physical hunger arises gradually and can be satisfied with a balanced meal. Emotional hunger, on the other hand, tends to come on suddenly and is often linked to specific emotions or situations. Learning to identify and address emotional hunger can help prevent unnecessary cravings.

3. Plan Balanced Meals and Snacks: Maintaining stable blood sugar levels throughout the day can help reduce cravings and hunger pangs. Plan your meals and snacks in advance, ensuring they include a combination of protein, healthy fats, and fiber. These nutrients promote satiety and help keep you feeling fuller for longer.

4. Stay Hydrated: Thirst is often mistaken for hunger, leading to unnecessary cravings. Stay hydrated by drinking an adequate amount of water throughout the day. Aim for at least eight glasses of water or more, depending on your activity level and individual needs. Keeping hydrated can help reduce the frequency of cravings and promote a sense of fullness.

5. Incorporate Protein and Fiber: Including protein and fiber-rich foods in your meals can help control cravings and keep you satisfied. Protein-rich foods, such as lean meats, poultry, fish, eggs, tofu, and legumes, provide a feeling of fullness and help stabilize blood sugar levels. Fiber-rich foods, such as fruits, vegetables, whole grains, and legumes, also contribute to satiety and promote digestive health.

6. Mindful Eating: Practicing mindful eating can help you become more aware of your body's hunger and fullness cues. Take your time while eating, savoring each bite, and paying attention to the taste, texture, and aroma of your food. By eating slowly and mindfully, you give your body a chance to recognize when it is satisfied, reducing the likelihood of cravings.

7. Find Healthy Substitutes: If you have specific cravings for unhealthy foods, look for healthier alternatives that can satisfy your taste buds. For example, if you are craving something sweet, opt for a piece of fruit or a small serving of dark chocolate. If you desire something crunchy, reach for carrot sticks or air-popped popcorn instead of chips. Experiment with nutritious substitutes that can help curb cravings without derailing your healthy eating plan.

8. Manage Stress: Stress can trigger cravings and emotional eating. Find healthy ways to manage stress, such as engaging in regular exercise, practicing relaxation techniques like deep breathing or yoga, or pursuing activities you enjoy. By reducing stress levels, you can minimize the likelihood of turning to food for comfort or distraction.

9. Get Enough Sleep: Inadequate sleep can disrupt hunger and satiety hormones, leading to increased cravings. Aim for seven to nine hours of quality sleep each night to support your overall well-being. Prioritize a consistent sleep schedule and create a relaxing bedtime routine to improve the quality and duration of your sleep.

10. Seek Professional Help if Needed: If you find it challenging to manage cravings and hunger pangs on your own, consider seeking support from a registered dietitian or a healthcare professional specializing in nutrition. They can provide personalized guidance and strategies tailored to your specific needs and goals.

Remember, managing cravings and hunger pangs is a journey that requires patience and self-compassion. By implementing these strategies and adopting a mindful approach to eating, you can develop a healthier relationship with food and better manage your cravings.

Navigating Social Situations and Dining Out

Social situations and dining out can present challenges when you're trying to maintain a healthy lifestyle or follow a specific dietary plan. However, with some planning and mindful choices, you can successfully navigate these situations while still enjoying social interactions and delicious meals.

1. Plan Ahead: Before heading to a social gathering or restaurant, take some time to plan ahead. If possible, check the menu in advance to identify healthier options or dishes that align with your dietary preferences. This way, you can make informed choices and avoid feeling overwhelmed when you arrive.

2. Communicate Your Needs: If you have specific dietary restrictions or preferences, don't be afraid to communicate them to your host or the restaurant staff. Most establishments are accommodating and willing to make modifications to suit your needs. By clearly expressing your requirements, you can ensure that there are suitable options available for you.

3. Fill Up on Nutrient-Dense Foods: Prior to attending a social event or going out for a meal, try to have a balanced and nutritious snack or meal. By filling up on foods that are rich in nutrients, such as fruits, vegetables, lean proteins, and whole grains, you can help curb excessive hunger and make better choices when faced with tempting options.

4. Practice Portion Control: While dining out, portion sizes can often be larger than what you need. Be mindful of portion sizes and consider sharing a dish with a friend or opting for a smaller-sized portion. If leftovers are allowed, pack them up to enjoy later instead of feeling compelled to finish everything on your plate.

5. Be Mindful of Hidden Ingredients: Some dishes or foods may contain hidden ingredients that may not align with your dietary preferences or restrictions. Be mindful of sauces, dressings, or added sugars that may be present in certain dishes. If unsure, don't hesitate to ask the restaurant staff about the ingredients or how the food is prepared.

6. Make Smart Menu Choices: When browsing through the menu, look for options that are prepared using healthier cooking methods such as grilling, baking, or steaming. Choose dishes that are rich in vegetables, lean proteins, and whole grains. Opt for sauces or dressings on the side so that you can control the amount you consume.

7. Focus on Enjoyment and Socializing: While it's important to be mindful of your food choices, remember that social situations are also about enjoying the company and the experience. Instead of solely focusing on the food, engage in conversations, savor the moment, and make lasting memories with friends and loved ones.

8. Stay Hydrated: Drinking water throughout the meal can help you stay hydrated and potentially reduce overeating. Sip water between bites and pay attention to your body's signals of hunger and fullness.

9. Practice Moderation, Not Deprivation: It's essential to strike a balance between enjoying your favorite foods and maintaining a healthy lifestyle. Allow yourself to indulge in moderation, savoring the flavors and enjoying the experience. Avoid an all-or-nothing mindset, as this can lead to feelings of guilt or deprivation.

10. Be Kind to Yourself: Remember that occasional indulgences or deviations from your usual eating pattern are normal and part of a balanced approach to food. If you do indulge more than intended, practice self-compassion and avoid dwelling on feelings of guilt. Instead, focus on making healthier choices moving forward.

Navigating social situations and dining out can be challenging, but with a proactive mindset and mindful decision-making, you can enjoy the experience while staying true to your health goals. Remember that flexibility and balance are key, and finding joy in both the food and the company is paramount.

Staying Motivated And Accountable

Maintaining motivation and accountability is essential when striving to achieve personal or professional goals. However, it is not always easy to stay on track and consistently put in the necessary effort. In this section, we will explore some strategies to help you stay motivated and accountable.

1. Set Clear and Realistic Goals: Start by defining your goals clearly. Make them specific, measurable, achievable, relevant, and time-bound (SMART). When your goals are well-defined, it becomes easier to stay motivated because you have a clear target to work towards. Ensure that your goals are also realistic, taking into account your abilities, resources, and time constraints.

2. Find Your Why: Understanding your motivation behind your goals can provide a powerful driving force. Reflect on why you want to achieve these goals and how they align with your values and aspirations. When you have a strong emotional connection to your goals, it becomes easier to stay motivated and focused, even when faced with challenges.

3. Break It Down: Large goals can sometimes feel overwhelming, leading to a lack of motivation. Break your goals down into smaller, manageable tasks or milestones. This allows you to experience a sense of progress and accomplishment along the way, boosting your motivation. Celebrate each milestone achieved, and use it as an opportunity to reassess and adjust your approach if needed.

4. Visualize Success: Create a vivid mental image of what success looks like for you. Visualizing your goals as already achieved can increase your motivation and make them feel more attainable. Imagine the positive impact achieving your goals will have on your life and use this visualization as a source of inspiration during challenging times.

5. Stay Positive and Practice Self-Compassion: It's natural to face setbacks and encounter obstacles on your journey. Instead of being hard on yourself, practice self-compassion and focus on learning from mistakes. Surround yourself with positive influences, whether it's supportive friends, inspiring books, or motivational podcasts. Cultivating a positive mindset can help you maintain motivation and overcome challenges more effectively.

6. Find an Accountability Partner: Share your goals and progress with someone you trust, such as a friend, family member, or mentor. Having an accountability partner can provide encouragement, support, and an external perspective on your progress. Regular check-ins with your accountability partner can help you stay on track and make adjustments if necessary.

7. Create a Routine: Establishing a routine can help you develop consistent habits and make progress towards your goals. Set aside dedicated time each day or week to work on specific tasks related to your goals. By making your goals a priority in your schedule, you are more likely to stay motivated and hold yourself accountable.

8. Use Rewards and Incentives: Celebrating milestones and rewarding yourself along the way can boost motivation and provide a sense of accomplishment. Consider setting up a reward system where you treat yourself after achieving certain goals or completing specific tasks. These rewards can serve as additional motivation and reinforce positive behaviors.

Remember, staying motivated and accountable is a continuous process. Be flexible and willing to adapt your strategies as you progress. Regularly reassess your goals, track your progress, and make adjustments to your approach if needed. By implementing these strategies, you can increase your chances of staying motivated and achieving your desired outcomes.

Establishing A Support System

Having a support system in place can significantly enhance your ability to achieve your goals, navigate challenges, and maintain motivation. A support system provides encouragement, advice, and accountability, helping you stay on track and overcome obstacles. Here are some steps to establish an effective support system:

1. Identify Your Needs: Reflect on the areas where you would benefit from support. Are you looking for emotional encouragement, practical advice, or accountability? Understanding your specific needs will help you identify the types of individuals or resources that would make up an effective support system.

2. Reach Out to Friends and Family: Start by reaching out to your friends and family members who are supportive and understanding. Share your goals and aspirations with them, and explain why their support is important to you. Having loved ones who believe in you and cheer you on can be a great source of motivation and encouragement.

3. Join a Community or Group: Seek out communities or groups that share your interests or goals. This could be a professional network, an online forum, a local meetup group, or even a social media group. Engage with others who have similar ambitions and challenges, as they can provide valuable insights, advice, and empathy.

4. Find a Mentor or Coach: Consider finding a mentor or coach who has experience in the areas you are pursuing.

A mentor can offer guidance, share their knowledge, and provide valuable feedback. They can help you stay accountable and push you to reach your full potential. Look for mentors who align with your values and goals, and establish a regular cadence for communication and support.

5. Seek Professional Support: Depending on your goals, it may be beneficial to seek professional support. For example, if you're working on personal development or mental health goals, you might consider consulting a therapist or counselor. They can provide specialized guidance and support tailored to your specific needs.

6. Attend Workshops or Classes: Explore workshops, classes, or seminars related to your goals or interests. These can be excellent opportunities to meet like-minded individuals, learn from experts, and expand your network. Engaging in these learning experiences can not only provide valuable knowledge but also connect you with individuals who can offer ongoing support.

7. Participate in Accountability Groups: Join or create an accountability group with individuals who have similar goals. Accountability groups typically meet regularly to share progress, discuss challenges, and hold each other accountable. This collective support can foster a sense of community and provide an additional layer of motivation.

8. Utilize Online Resources: Take advantage of the numerous online resources available to support your goals. Online forums, blogs, podcasts, and social media communities can offer valuable insights, motivation, and connections. Engage actively in these online spaces, contribute to discussions, and seek advice from experts in your field.

Remember that establishing a support system is a two-way street. Be willing to offer support, encouragement, and accountability to others in return. Building strong relationships within your support system requires mutual trust, respect, and active engagement.

Tracking Progress And Celebrating Milestones

Tracking your progress and celebrating milestones along the way can be powerful motivators on your journey towards achieving your goals. They provide a sense of accomplishment, reinforce positive behaviors, and help you stay focused. Here are some strategies for effectively tracking progress and celebrating milestones:

1. Define Measurable Milestones: Break down your goals into smaller, measurable milestones. These milestones should be specific and tangible, allowing you to track your progress accurately. For example, if your goal is to lose weight, you can set milestones based on the number of pounds lost or inches reduced.

2. Use a Visual Tracker: Create a visual representation of your progress using charts, graphs, or a habit tracker. This allows you to see your progress at a glance and provides a visual reminder of how far you've come. Place your visual tracker somewhere visible, such as on your desk or fridge, to serve as a daily reminder of your goals.

3. Set Deadlines and Timelines: Establish deadlines and timelines for your milestones. Having a specific timeframe creates a sense of urgency and helps you stay focused. It also provides a benchmark against which you can measure your progress. Make sure your deadlines are realistic and achievable, taking into account any potential challenges or obstacles that may arise.

4. Track Quantitative and Qualitative Data: When monitoring your progress, consider both quantitative and qualitative data. Quantitative data includes measurable metrics such as the number of tasks completed, revenue generated, or hours invested. Qualitative data focuses on subjective aspects, such as the quality of your work or the satisfaction you feel towards your progress. By tracking both types of data, you can gain a holistic understanding of your achievements.

5. Use Technology and Apps: Leverage technology and apps designed for progress tracking. There are numerous productivity and goal-tracking apps available that can help you monitor your milestones, track habits, and provide reminders. These apps often offer features like progress charts, goal reminders, and notifications to keep you on track.

6. Regularly Review and Reflect: Schedule regular check-ins to review your progress and reflect on your achievements. This can be done weekly, monthly, or at any interval that works best for you. Take the time to assess your performance, identify areas for improvement, and make adjustments to your strategies if needed. Reflecting on your progress can also reinforce your motivation and provide a sense of direction.

7. Celebrate Milestones: Celebrate your achievements and milestones along the way. Recognize the effort you've put in and reward yourself for reaching significant milestones. Celebrations can take various forms, such as treating yourself to something you enjoy, taking a day off, or sharing your success with friends and family. Celebrating milestones boosts morale, reinforces positive behaviors, and keeps you motivated on your journey.

8. Learn from Setbacks: Acknowledge that setbacks and obstacles are a natural part of any journey. Instead of getting discouraged, use setbacks as opportunities for growth and learning. When faced with challenges, analyze what went wrong, identify lessons learned, and adjust your strategies accordingly. By embracing setbacks as learning experiences, you can continue to make progress and stay motivated.

Remember that tracking progress and celebrating milestones are not just about the destination but also about the journey itself. Enjoy the process, celebrate every step forward, and use your progress as fuel to keep moving towards your goals.

In conclusion, staying motivated and accountable requires a combination of strategies, such as setting clear goals, finding support, tracking progress, and celebrating milestones. By implementing these approaches, you can enhance your chances of success and maintain a positive mindset throughout your journey. Remember to stay flexible, adapt as needed, and celebrate the small victories along the way.

Incorporating Exercise Into The Zone Program

The Zone program is a popular approach to nutrition and overall wellness that focuses on balancing macronutrients to achieve optimal health and performance. While nutrition plays a crucial role in The Zone program, incorporating exercise is equally important to maximize its benefits. Exercise not only helps with weight management but also enhances cardiovascular health, boosts mood, and improves overall well-being.

1. Understanding The Zone program: Before incorporating exercise into The Zone program, it's essential to have a clear understanding of its principles. The Zone program emphasizes the consumption of balanced meals that include a specific ratio of proteins, carbohydrates, and fats. The goal is to stabilize blood sugar levels, control inflammation, and maintain hormonal balance. By understanding the fundamental principles of The Zone program, you can align your exercise routine with its goals.

2. Choosing the right exercises: The type of exercises you choose should complement The Zone program and support its objectives. Aim for a combination of cardiovascular exercises, strength training, and flexibility exercises. Cardiovascular exercises such as running, swimming, or cycling can improve your endurance, burn calories, and enhance cardiovascular health. Strength training exercises like weightlifting or bodyweight exercises can help build muscle mass, increase metabolism, and improve body composition. Don't forget to include flexibility exercises like stretching or yoga to improve joint mobility and prevent injuries.

3. Timing of exercise sessions: Incorporating exercise into The Zone program requires thoughtful planning regarding the timing of your workouts. Consider scheduling your exercise sessions at a time when you have the most energy and motivation. Some individuals prefer exercising in the morning, while others find it more convenient in the afternoon or evening. Experiment with different timings to identify what works best for you. Remember that consistency is key, so try to establish a regular exercise routine that aligns with your daily schedule.

4. Balancing exercise intensity: When incorporating exercise into The Zone program, it's important to balance the intensity of your workouts. Moderate-intensity exercises, such as brisk walking or cycling at a moderate pace, can help improve cardiovascular fitness without excessively taxing the body. High-intensity interval training (HIIT) is also a valuable option as it combines short bursts of intense exercise with recovery periods. HIIT can be an effective way to burn calories, improve metabolic function, and stimulate fat loss. However, it's crucial to listen to your body and avoid overtraining, as excessive exercise can lead to burnout and hinder progress.

5. Recovery and rest days: Incorporating exercise into The Zone program should also prioritize rest and recovery days. Rest days are essential for allowing your body to repair and adapt to the physical stress of exercise. It's during the recovery phase that your muscles grow stronger and more resilient. Additionally, sufficient rest helps prevent injuries and reduces the risk of overtraining. Aim to include at least one or two rest days per week in your exercise routine. On these days, focus on active recovery activities like stretching or light yoga.

6. Tracking progress: To ensure that exercise is effectively incorporated into The Zone program, tracking your progress is vital. Keep a record of your workouts, including the type of exercises, duration, and intensity. You can also track other metrics such as heart rate, distance covered, or weight lifted. By monitoring your progress, you can assess your improvement over time, identify areas that need adjustment, and stay motivated. There are various fitness apps and wearables available that can assist you in tracking and analyzing your exercise data.

Incorporating exercise into The Zone program offers numerous benefits, and by following these guidelines, you can optimize your fitness journey while aligning it with the principles of The Zone program. Remember to consult with a healthcare professional or a certified fitness trainer before starting any new exercise program, especially if you have any pre-existing medical conditions or concerns.

Incorporating exercise into The Zone program offers numerous benefits that go beyond weight management. Regular physical activity has a wide range of positive effects on both physical and mental health. Let's explore some of the key benefits:

1. **Weight management:** Exercise plays a crucial role in maintaining a healthy weight and body composition. It helps burn calories and build muscle mass, which increases metabolism and contributes to weight loss or weight maintenance. By incorporating exercise into The Zone program, you can enhance your ability to achieve and maintain your desired weight.

2. **Cardiovascular health:** Engaging in regular cardiovascular exercises, such as running, swimming, or cycling, improves heart health and lowers the risk of cardiovascular diseases. It strengthens the heart muscle, improves circulation, and enhances the efficiency of oxygen and nutrient delivery throughout the body. By incorporating cardiovascular exercises into your Zone program, you can improve your overall cardiovascular

fitness.

3. Increased energy levels: Regular physical activity has been shown to boost energy levels and combat feelings of fatigue. Exercise improves blood flow and oxygen delivery to the muscles and tissues, promoting alertness and vitality. By incorporating exercise into The Zone program, you can experience increased energy levels throughout the day, enhancing your productivity and overall well-being.

4. Mood enhancement: Exercise has powerful mood-enhancing effects. Physical activity stimulates the release of endorphins, which are neurotransmitters responsible for promoting feelings of happiness and reducing stress and anxiety. Regular exercise can improve mood, alleviate symptoms of depression, and enhance overall mental well-being. By incorporating exercise into The Zone program, you can support your emotional health and promote a positive mindset.

5. Improved cognitive function: Physical activity has been shown to have positive effects on cognitive function and brain health. Exercise promotes blood flow to the brain, stimulates the growth of new neurons, and enhances memory, attention, and problem-solving abilities. By incorporating exercise into The Zone program, you can optimize your cognitive function and support long-term brain health.

6. Stronger immune system: Regular physical activity has been linked to a stronger immune system. Exercise enhances the circulation of immune cells and antibodies, which helps the body fight off infections and diseases. By incorporating exercise into The Zone program, you can strengthen your immune system and reduce the risk of illness.

7. Better sleep quality: Engaging in regular exercise has been shown to improve sleep quality and duration. Physical activity helps regulate the sleep-wake cycle, promotes relaxation, and reduces symptoms of insomnia. By incorporating exercise into The Zone program, you can experience more restful and rejuvenating sleep, allowing your body to recover and recharge.

8. Increased longevity: Regular physical activity is associated with a longer and healthier lifespan. Studies have shown that individuals who engage in regular exercise have a reduced risk of chronic diseases such as heart disease, diabetes, and certain types of cancer. By incorporating exercise into The Zone program, you can contribute to a longer and more vibrant life.

Finding the right workout routine for your goals is essential to ensure that you enjoy the benefits of regular physical activity. Consider your personal preferences, fitness level, and specific objectives when selecting a workout routine. Whether it's strength training, cardiovascular exercises, or a combination of various activities, the key is to find a routine that you find enjoyable and sustainable. Consult with a fitness professional or personal trainer if needed to create a personalized workout plan that aligns with The Zone program and helps you achieve your fitness goals.

CHAPTER FIVE

Fine-Tuning Your Zone Experience

Personalizing The Zone

Personalizing The Zone is a concept that involves tailoring your environment, routines, and habits to optimize your productivity, well-being, and overall satisfaction. The idea behind personalizing the zone is to create an environment that supports your goals, preferences, and individual needs. By understanding yourself and making intentional adjustments, you can enhance your performance and make the most out of your time and resources.

One way to personalize the zone is by customizing your physical environment. Your surroundings can have a significant impact on your mood, focus, and creativity. Consider factors such as lighting, temperature, noise levels, and organization when setting up your workspace or living area. Experiment with different arrangements and find what works best for you. Some people thrive in a minimalist environment, while others find inspiration in a more vibrant and eclectic setting. **Identify the elements that positively influence your mindset and productivity,**

and incorporate them into your space.

Another aspect of personalizing the zone is adapting your routines and habits to suit your unique needs. Everyone has different energy levels, preferences, and peak performance times. **Pay attention to your natural rhythms and align your activities accordingly**. If you're a morning person, prioritize demanding tasks and creative work during those hours. If you find yourself more alert and focused after exercising, schedule your most challenging work sessions for the afternoon. By understanding your personal patterns, you can optimize your productivity and avoid burnout.

Additionally, personalizing the zone involves identifying and leveraging your strengths. Each person has unique skills, talents, and interests. By focusing on activities that align with your strengths, you can increase your motivation, engagement, and overall satisfaction. **Take some time to reflect on your passions and areas where you excel**. Consider how you can incorporate these strengths into your work or personal life. For example, if you have strong interpersonal skills, you might explore opportunities that involve teamwork or leadership. By maximizing your strengths, you can achieve better results and experience a greater sense of fulfillment.

Furthermore, personalizing the zone involves managing your energy and well-being. Recognize that you have limited mental and physical resources, and it's important to allocate them wisely. **Pay attention to your nutrition, sleep, and stress levels**. Adjust your diet to include macronutrient ratios that support your specific needs, which we will explore in the next topic. Ensure you're getting enough restful sleep to recharge and recover. Find healthy ways to manage stress, such as practicing mindfulness or engaging in regular physical activity. By taking care of your overall well-being, you'll have more energy and resilience to perform at your best.

Adjusting Macronutrient Ratios For Specific Needs

Macronutrients are the essential nutrients that provide energy and building blocks for our bodies. They include carbohydrates, proteins, and fats. While the overall macronutrient ratio remains important for a balanced diet, adjusting the macronutrient ratios for specific needs can have additional benefits depending on individual goals, health conditions, and lifestyle choices.

One common goal that often leads to adjusting macronutrient ratios is weight management. When aiming to lose weight, reducing the proportion of carbohydrates and increasing protein intake can be beneficial. Protein is known to promote satiety, which helps control hunger and prevent overeating. Additionally, it supports muscle maintenance and repair during weight loss, which can help preserve lean body mass. On the other hand, reducing the intake of carbohydrates, especially refined sugars and processed grains, can help regulate blood sugar levels and promote fat burning.

For individuals who are involved in intense physical training or have a high level of physical activity, adjusting macronutrient ratios can optimize performance and recovery. **Increasing the proportion of carbohydrates can provide the necessary fuel for sustained energy during exercise**. Carbohydrates are the primary source of energy for the body, and consuming an adequate amount can enhance endurance and prevent fatigue. However, it's important to focus on complex carbohydrates such as whole grains, fruits, and vegetables, which provide a steady release of energy and essential nutrients.

Athletes and individuals engaged in strength training may benefit from adjusting their macronutrient ratios to include a higher proportion of protein. Protein is crucial for muscle repair, growth, and recovery. Consuming an adequate amount of protein can help optimize muscle protein synthesis and enhance post-workout recovery. **A general guideline for athletes is to consume approximately 1.2-2.0 grams of protein per kilogram of body weight per day**, depending on the specific sport or activity level.

In some cases, individuals may have specific health conditions that require adjustments in macronutrient ratios. For example, individuals with diabetes may benefit from reducing the proportion of carbohydrates and focusing on consuming healthy fats and lean proteins. This approach can help regulate blood sugar levels and improve insulin sensitivity. Similarly, individuals with certain metabolic disorders may benefit from following a ketogenic diet, which is high in fats and very low in carbohydrates. This can help shift the body's metabolism to rely on fats for fuel.

It's important to note that when adjusting macronutrient ratios, it's essential to prioritize nutrient-dense foods and maintain a balanced diet. **Focusing on whole, unprocessed foods and paying attention to portion sizes is crucial**. While macronutrient ratios play a role in achieving specific goals, it's equally important to consider other aspects of nutrition, such as consuming an adequate amount of vitamins, minerals, and fiber.

In conclusion, adjusting macronutrient ratios for specific needs can have various benefits depending on individual goals, health conditions, and lifestyle choices. Whether it's for weight management, athletic performance, or managing certain health conditions, making intentional adjustments to the proportions of carbohydrates, proteins, and fats can optimize results. However, it's essential to prioritize nutrient-dense foods, maintain a balanced diet, and consult with a healthcare professional or registered dietitian for personalized guidance.

Understanding The Role Of Supplements

Supplements play a significant role in supporting overall health and well-being. They are designed to complement a balanced diet and provide additional nutrients that may be lacking in one's regular intake. While it's important to obtain essential nutrients from food sources, supplements can serve as a valuable addition to fill potential gaps and meet specific nutritional needs.

1. Enhancing Nutrient Intake: One of the primary purposes of supplements is to enhance nutrient intake. Even with a well-rounded diet, individuals may struggle to consume adequate amounts of certain vitamins, minerals, or other essential compounds. Supplements can bridge this gap and ensure the body receives the necessary nutrients for optimal functioning.

2. Addressing Deficiencies: Supplements are particularly beneficial for addressing nutrient deficiencies. Some individuals may have specific dietary restrictions or medical conditions that prevent them from obtaining sufficient nutrients through food alone. In such cases, targeted supplements can help correct deficiencies and prevent associated health issues.

3. Supporting Specialized Diets: Certain dietary approaches, such as veganism or vegetarianism, may require additional supplementation. For instance, individuals following a plant-based diet might need to supplement with vitamin B12, which is predominantly found in animal products. Similarly, pregnant women often require extra folic acid to support fetal development.

4. Promoting Specific Health Goals: Supplements can also be used to promote specific health goals. For example, athletes or individuals engaging in intense physical activity may benefit from supplements that support muscle recovery, such as protein or branched-chain amino acids. Similarly, individuals aiming for healthy hair, skin, and nails may opt for supplements containing biotin or collagen.

5. Compensating for Lifestyle Factors: Modern lifestyles, such as high stress levels or frequent travel, can impact nutrient absorption and utilization. Supplements can help compensate for these factors by providing the body with extra support. Adaptogenic herbs like ashwagandha or Rhodiola rosea are commonly used to manage stress, while probiotics can help maintain gut health during travel or antibiotic use.

While supplements offer various benefits, it's essential to approach their use with caution. Consulting with a healthcare professional is highly recommended to determine the most appropriate and safe supplement regimen based on individual needs and health conditions.

Exploring Recommended Supplements For The Zone

The Zone diet, developed by Dr. Barry Sears, emphasizes balancing macronutrient ratios to promote optimal hormonal balance and weight management. This dietary approach recommends a specific distribution of carbohydrates, proteins, and fats, aiming to maintain stable blood sugar levels and reduce inflammation. While the Zone diet primarily focuses on food choices, certain supplements can support its principles and enhance overall results.

1. Omega-3 Fatty Acids: Omega-3 fatty acids, commonly found in fish oil supplements, are recommended for individuals following The Zone diet. These essential fats offer anti-inflammatory benefits and support cardiovascular health. Omega-3 supplementation can help individuals achieve the recommended balance of fats while providing additional health advantages.

2. Antioxidants: Antioxidant supplements, such as vitamins C and E, can complement The Zone diet by reducing oxidative stress and inflammation. These nutrients scavenge free radicals, which can damage cells and contribute to chronic diseases. Including antioxidant-rich supplements can further support the anti-inflammatory aspect of The Zone diet.

3. Probiotics: The Zone diet encourages gut health, as the balance of good bacteria in the digestive system can influence overall well-being. Probiotic supplements containing beneficial strains like Lactobacillus and Bifidobacterium can enhance digestion, support immune function, and contribute to a healthy gut microbiome.

4. Chromium: Chromium is a mineral that plays a role in regulating blood sugar levels and insulin sensitivity. The Zone diet aims to maintain stable blood sugar levels, and supplementing with chromium may further support this goal. By improving insulin function, chromium can help enhance carbohydrate metabolism and potentially aid in weight management.

5. Magnesium: Magnesium is an essential mineral involved in numerous bodily functions, including energy production and muscle function. The Zone diet encourages consuming magnesium-rich foods, such as leafy greens and nuts. However, some individuals may benefit from magnesium supplementation to ensure adequate intake and support overall well-being.

6. B vitamins: B vitamins, including B6, B12, and folate, are crucial for energy production, metabolism, and nerve function. While The Zone diet emphasizes whole foods rich in B vitamins, certain individuals may require supplementation. For instance, vegetarians or individuals with specific genetic variations that affect B vitamin absorption may benefit from additional supplementation.

It's important to note that while these supplements may support The Zone diet principles, they should not be considered a substitute for a balanced diet. Whole, nutrient-dense foods remain the foundation of this dietary approach. Before incorporating any supplements into The Zone diet, it is advisable to consult with a healthcare professional or registered dietitian to ensure their suitability and proper dosages.

Consulting With A Healthcare Professional

When considering dietary changes, incorporating supplements, or addressing specific health concerns, consulting with a healthcare professional is crucial. Healthcare professionals, such as doctors, registered dietitians, or nutritionists, possess the expertise to provide personalized guidance and recommendations based on an individual's unique circumstances. Here are a few reasons why consulting with a healthcare professional is important:

1. Personalized Advice: Healthcare professionals can assess an individual's health history, lifestyle factors, and specific needs to provide personalized advice. They can tailor dietary recommendations and supplement regimens to meet individual goals and optimize overall well-being.

2. Safety and Compatibility: Healthcare professionals can evaluate the safety and compatibility of supplements with medications, pre-existing conditions, or specific dietary requirements. They can identify potential interactions or contraindications that may pose risks to an individual's health.

3. Evidence-Based Guidance: Healthcare professionals stay up-to-date with the latest research and evidence in nutrition and supplementation. They can provide evidence-based guidance and recommendations, ensuring individuals make informed choices based on reliable information.

4. Monitoring and Follow-Up: Consulting with a healthcare professional allows for ongoing monitoring and follow-up. They can track progress, assess any changes in health status, and make necessary adjustments to the supplement regimen or dietary plan as needed.

5. Addressing Underlying Issues: Healthcare professionals are trained to identify underlying health issues or nutrient deficiencies that may require further investigation or treatment. They can conduct thorough assessments, order diagnostic tests if necessary, and provide appropriate interventions beyond supplements alone.

Troubleshooting Common Issues

Troubleshooting common issues is an essential skill to have, whether it's in your personal or professional life. In various situations, problems may arise that require a systematic approach to identify the root cause and implement effective solutions. This section will delve into some common issues that individuals encounter and provide guidance on how to troubleshoot them effectively.

1. Connectivity problems in a network: One of the most common issues people encounter is connectivity problems in their network. When troubleshooting such issues, it is crucial to follow a step-by-step process. First, check if the cables are properly connected and ensure there are no physical damages. Next, restart the modem and router to refresh the network connection. If the problem persists, check the network settings on your device and verify that the correct network name and password are entered. Additionally, running a diagnostic test on the network can help identify any underlying issues.

2. Software crashes: Dealing with software crashes can be frustrating, but troubleshooting techniques can help resolve these issues. Start by restarting the computer and relaunching the software. If the problem persists, check for any available software updates and install them. It is also helpful to disable any recently installed plugins or extensions, as they may be causing conflicts. Clearing the cache and temporary files can also help resolve crashes. If none of these steps work, uninstalling and reinstalling the software might be necessary.

3. Printer problems: Printer issues can disrupt productivity, but troubleshooting can help overcome them. Begin by checking the connection between the printer and the computer or network. Ensure that the printer is powered on and there are no paper jams. If the printer is connected wirelessly, verify that it is connected to the correct network. Additionally, updating the printer drivers can often resolve compatibility issues. If the problem persists, restarting both the printer and the computer can sometimes solve the issue.

4. Slow computer performance: A slow computer can be a hindrance to efficient work. To troubleshoot this issue, start by checking the available storage space on the computer's hard drive. Delete unnecessary files and programs to free up space. Running a virus scan can also identify and remove any malware that might be slowing down the system. Another potential solution is to increase the computer's RAM capacity, as insufficient memory can lead to performance issues. Additionally, disabling unnecessary startup programs and optimizing the computer's settings can help improve its speed.

5. Battery drain on mobile devices: Many individuals experience rapid battery drain on their mobile devices. To troubleshoot this issue, first, check for any software updates and install them, as updates often include battery optimization improvements. Adjusting the screen brightness to a lower setting and enabling power-saving mode can also conserve battery life. Closing unnecessary background apps and disabling features like Bluetooth and location services when not in use can further extend battery life. If the battery drain issue persists, it might be worth considering a battery replacement.

Addressing Plateaus And Weight Loss Stalls

Addressing plateaus and weight loss stalls is a common challenge faced by individuals on a weight loss journey. It can be frustrating when progress comes to a halt despite consistent efforts. However, with the right approach, plateaus can be overcome. The following strategies can help address plateaus and promote continued weight loss:

1. Review and adjust your calorie intake: When weight loss stalls, it may be necessary to reassess your calorie intake. As you lose weight, your body's energy needs may decrease, so you may need to consume fewer calories to continue losing weight. Consider tracking your food intake and ensuring you are in a calorie deficit. Gradually reducing your calorie intake by a small amount can jumpstart weight loss again without causing excessive restriction.

2. Vary your exercise routine: Plateaus can occur when your body adapts to a specific exercise routine. To overcome this, it's important to introduce variety into your workouts. Incorporate different types of exercises, such as cardio, strength training, and flexibility exercises. Try new activities like swimming, cycling, or dance classes. Changing the intensity, duration, and frequency of your workouts can also stimulate your body and kickstart weight loss. Additionally, consider working with a personal trainer who can design a tailored workout plan to challenge your body and break through the plateau.

3. Monitor portion sizes and food quality: Sometimes, weight loss stalls because we unknowingly consume more calories than we realize. Take a closer look at your portion sizes and ensure they align with your weight loss goals. Use measuring cups or a food scale to accurately measure your food. Additionally, focus on the quality of your diet. Incorporate nutrient-dense foods, such as fruits, vegetables, lean proteins, and whole grains, while minimizing processed and high-calorie foods. This can help optimize your nutrition and support continued weight loss.

4. Evaluate stress levels and sleep quality: High levels of stress and inadequate sleep can impact weight loss progress. When we're stressed, our bodies produce cortisol, a hormone that can contribute to weight gain or hinder weight loss. Similarly, poor sleep affects our metabolism and hormone regulation. Take time to manage stress through relaxation techniques, such as meditation, deep breathing exercises, or engaging in activities you enjoy. Aim for at least 7-8 hours of quality sleep each night. Prioritizing stress reduction and sufficient sleep can positively impact weight loss efforts.

5. Stay consistent and patient: Weight loss plateaus are a normal part of the journey, and it's essential to remain consistent and patient during these times. Remember that weight loss is not linear, and everyone's body responds differently. Focus on other positive changes in your health, such as increased energy levels, improved fitness, and overall well-being. Stay committed to your healthy habits and trust the process. With time and persistence, you are likely to break through the plateau and continue progressing towards your weight loss goals.

Managing Energy Fluctuations

Managing energy fluctuations is crucial for maintaining

productivity, overall well-being, and a balanced lifestyle. Energy levels can fluctuate throughout the day, and understanding how to manage these fluctuations can help optimize performance and enhance quality of life. Here are some strategies to effectively manage energy fluctuations:

1. Establish a consistent sleep routine: Quality sleep is vital for maintaining optimal energy levels. Establish a regular sleep schedule by going to bed and waking up at the same time each day, even on weekends. Create a sleep-friendly environment by ensuring your bedroom is dark, quiet, and at a comfortable temperature. Avoid stimulating activities, such as using electronic devices or consuming caffeine, close to bedtime. Prioritizing good sleep hygiene can significantly improve energy levels throughout the day.

2. Eat balanced meals and snacks: Proper nutrition plays a crucial role in managing energy fluctuations. Focus on consuming balanced meals that include a combination of complex carbohydrates, lean proteins, and healthy fats. These nutrients provide sustained energy and help prevent blood sugar spikes and crashes. Incorporate regular healthy snacks between meals to maintain steady energy levels. Opt for whole foods, such as fruits, vegetables, nuts, and seeds, which provide essential nutrients and promote long-lasting energy.

3. Stay hydrated: Dehydration can lead to fatigue and decreased energy levels. Make sure to drink an adequate amount of water throughout the day to stay hydrated. Keep a water bottle with you and sip water regularly, especially during physical activity or when exposed to hot weather. If you struggle with drinking plain water, infuse it with fruits or herbs to add flavor. Additionally, limit your consumption of sugary beverages and alcohol, as they can contribute to dehydration and energy fluctuations.

4. Incorporate regular physical activity: Engaging in regular physical activity can help boost energy levels and overall well-being. Find activities that you enjoy and make them a part of your routine. Aim for at least 150 minutes of moderate-intensity aerobic exercise or 75 minutes of vigorous-intensity exercise per week, along with strength training exercises twice a week. Regular exercise not only enhances energy levels but also improves mood, reduces stress, and promotes better sleep.

5. Practice stress management techniques: Chronic stress can drain your energy reserves. It's essential to incorporate stress management techniques into your daily routine. Find activities that help you relax and unwind, such as practicing mindfulness or deep breathing exercises, engaging in hobbies, spending time in nature, or engaging in activities that bring you joy. Prioritizing self-care and managing stress effectively can help maintain consistent energy levels and improve overall well-being.

6. Prioritize breaks and rest: Taking regular breaks throughout the day and allowing yourself adequate rest is crucial for managing energy fluctuations. Avoid pushing yourself to the point of exhaustion. Incorporate short breaks during work or study sessions to recharge and refocus. Engage in activities that help you relax and rejuvenate, such as taking a short walk, listening to music, or practicing meditation. Additionally, ensure you have sufficient downtime and quality sleep to allow your body and mind to recover and recharge.

7. Identify and manage energy-draining factors: Pay attention to factors that drain your energy and take steps to manage or eliminate them. This can include minimizing exposure to negative influences, setting boundaries in personal and professional relationships, and learning to delegate tasks when possible. It's important to prioritize activities and responsibilities that align with your values and goals, allowing you to conserve energy for what truly matters to you.

By implementing these strategies, you can effectively manage energy fluctuations, maintain optimal energy levels, and enhance your overall well-being. Remember that everyone's energy patterns are unique, so it's essential to listen to your body, experiment with different approaches, and find what works best for you. With a balanced approach to managing energy, you can lead a more productive and fulfilling life.

CHAPTER SIX

Embracing The Zone As A Lifestyle

The Zone diet, developed by Dr. Barry Sears, is a popular dietary approach that emphasizes balancing macronutrients to achieve optimal hormonal balance in the body. It promotes a balance of carbohydrates, proteins, and fats in each meal to control insulin levels and promote overall well-being. While many people initially adopt the Zone diet as a temporary way to achieve specific health or weight goals, embracing it as a lifestyle can bring about long-term benefits.

1. Mindful Meal Planning

One of the key principles of the Zone diet is mindful meal planning. Instead of simply focusing on calorie counting or restricting certain food groups, the Zone encourages individuals to build a balanced plate consisting of lean proteins, carbohydrates, and healthy fats. By planning meals in advance and ensuring each one adheres to this balance, individuals can establish a sustainable and nourishing eating routine.

2. Controlling Insulin Levels

The Zone diet places particular emphasis on controlling insulin levels in the body. Insulin, a hormone produced by the pancreas, regulates blood sugar levels. When insulin levels are high, it can lead to increased fat storage and potential health issues such as obesity and diabetes. By following the Zone diet, which advocates for a controlled release of insulin through balanced meals, individuals can achieve better metabolic stability and improved overall health.

3. Steady Energy Levels

One of the benefits of embracing the Zone as a lifestyle is the potential for steady energy levels throughout the day. By consuming balanced meals that contain the right combination of macronutrients, individuals can avoid energy crashes and maintain a consistent level of focus and productivity. This can be especially beneficial for those with demanding work schedules or active lifestyles.

4. Enhanced Athletic Performance

For athletes or individuals who engage in regular physical activity, embracing the Zone as a lifestyle can bring about enhanced performance. The balanced macronutrient distribution in the diet provides a steady supply of energy to support workouts and aid in recovery. By optimizing nutrient intake, individuals may experience increased endurance, improved muscle recovery, and overall better athletic performance.

5. Weight Management

While weight loss is a common goal for many people, the Zone diet focuses more on body composition and overall health than solely on the number on the scale. By adhering to the balanced macronutrient ratios prescribed by the Zone, individuals may experience better weight management in the long run. The diet promotes the preservation of lean muscle mass while reducing body fat, which can result in a healthier body composition.

6. Long-Term Health Benefits

Embracing the Zone as a lifestyle can have numerous long-term health benefits. The balanced macronutrient ratios and focus on controlling insulin levels can contribute to improved heart health, reduced risk of chronic diseases, and better overall metabolic function. By adopting a sustainable approach to eating and making the Zone principles a part of one's daily life, individuals can work towards achieving lasting health benefits.

In conclusion, while the Zone diet is often viewed as a temporary approach for achieving specific health or weight goals, embracing it as a lifestyle can bring about sustainable changes and lasting results. By practicing mindful meal planning, controlling insulin levels, and reaping the benefits of steady energy levels, enhanced athletic performance, weight management, and long-term health benefits, individuals can transform the Zone diet into a holistic lifestyle that promotes overall well-being.

Moving Beyond A Temporary Diet Mindset

Many people approach diets with a temporary mindset, viewing them as a quick fix to achieve short-term goals such as weight loss or improved health. However, shifting the perspective from a temporary diet mindset to a long-term lifestyle approach can lead to more sustainable changes and lasting results. Rather than focusing on strict rules and restrictions, it's important to adopt a balanced and flexible approach to eating that can be maintained over time.

1. Cultivating a Mindset Shift

To move beyond a temporary diet mindset, it's crucial to cultivate a mindset shift. Instead of viewing a diet as a short-term solution, it's important to recognize that healthy eating is a lifelong commitment to nourishing the body and promoting overall well-being. Embracing the idea that food is fuel and a source of vitality can help shift the focus from restriction to nourishment.

2. Building Healthy Habits

A key aspect of transitioning to a long-term lifestyle approach is building healthy habits. Rather than relying on willpower alone, focus on creating sustainable routines and behaviors that support your health goals. This can include meal planning, mindful eating, regular physical activity, and finding ways to enjoy a variety of nutritious foods. By consistently practicing these habits, they can become ingrained and part of your daily life.

3. Finding Balance and Flexibility

A temporary diet often involves strict rules and restrictions that can be difficult to maintain in the long run. Instead, aim for a balanced and flexible approach to eating. Allow yourself to enjoy a wide variety of foods in moderation, including occasional treats, while also prioritizing nutrient-dense options. Incorporate a range of fruits, vegetables, whole grains, lean proteins, and healthy fats into your meals to ensure you're getting a diverse array of nutrients.

4. Mindful Eating

Practicing mindful eating is a powerful tool in moving beyond a temporary diet mindset. By being present and attentive to the eating experience, you can cultivate a greater awareness of hunger and fullness cues, as well as your body's individual needs. Pay attention to the flavors, textures, and satisfaction level of your meals. Eating slowly and savoring each bite can help you feel more satisfied and prevent overeating.

5. Emphasizing Progress over Perfection

It's important to shift the focus from perfection to progress when adopting a long-term lifestyle approach. Recognize that there will be ups and downs along the way, and that small steps forward are still steps in the right direction. Avoid getting caught up in all-or-nothing thinking and practice self-compassion. Celebrate your successes and learn from any setbacks, using them as opportunities for growth and adjustment.

6. Seeking Support and Accountability

Transitioning to a long-term lifestyle approach is often easier when you have support and accountability. Consider enlisting the help of a registered dietitian, joining a support group, or involving friends and family in your journey. Surrounding yourself with like-minded individuals who share similar goals can provide motivation, encouragement, and a sense of community.

In conclusion, moving beyond a temporary diet mindset involves shifting your perspective from a short-term fix to a long-term lifestyle approach. By cultivating a mindset shift, building healthy habits, finding balance and flexibility, practicing mindful eating, emphasizing progress over perfection, and seeking support and accountability, you can make sustainable changes that lead to lasting results. Remember that adopting a healthy lifestyle is a journey, and the focus should be on nourishing your body and prioritizing overall well-being for the long term.

Making Sustainable Changes For Lasting Results

When it comes to improving health and well-being, making sustainable changes is key. Instead of seeking quick fixes or following fad diets, focusing on long-term habits can lead to lasting results. Sustainable changes involve adopting healthy behaviors that can be maintained over time, promoting overall wellness and preventing the cycle of yo-yo dieting. By implementing the following strategies, individuals can establish a foundation for lasting success.

1. Set Realistic Goals

To make sustainable changes, it's important to set realistic and achievable goals. Setting goals that are too extreme or unrealistic can lead to frustration and discouragement. Instead, focus on smaller, attainable milestones that can be reached over time. Celebrate each achievement along the way, as this helps to maintain motivation and build confidence.

2. Gradual Progression

Rather than trying to overhaul your entire lifestyle overnight, focus on gradual progression. Start by making small changes to your daily routines and habits. For example, begin by incorporating more fruits and vegetables into your meals, increasing your water intake, or committing to a regular exercise routine. As these changes become ingrained, you can gradually add more healthy behaviors to your repertoire.

3. Prioritize Whole Foods

Making sustainable changes involves prioritizing whole, nutrient-dense foods. Whole foods, such as fruits, vegetables, whole grains, lean proteins, and healthy fats, provide essential nutrients and are generally lower in added sugars, sodium, and unhealthy fats. Aim to fill your plate with a variety of colors and textures, and experiment with different recipes and cooking methods to make healthy eating enjoyable and satisfying.

4. Practice Portion Control

Portion control plays a significant role in making sustainable changes. Even with healthy foods, consuming excessive amounts can hinder progress. It's important to be mindful of portion sizes and listen to your body's hunger and fullness cues. Consider using smaller plates and bowls, measuring food portions when needed, and taking the time to savor each bite. Mindful eating and paying attention to portion sizes can help prevent overeating and promote a healthier relationship with food.

5. Regular Physical Activity

Incorporating regular physical activity is essential for making sustainable changes. Find activities that you enjoy and that fit into your lifestyle, whether it's walking, jogging, dancing, swimming, or practicing yoga. Aim for at least 150 minutes of moderate-intensity aerobic activity per week, along with strength training exercises. Making physical activity a regular part of your routine not only supports weight management but also promotes overall health and well-being.

6. Focus on Consistency, Not Perfection

Consistency is key when it comes to making sustainable changes. Instead of striving for perfection, focus on progress and consistency over time. There may be days when you deviate from your plan or make choices that are not aligned with your goals, and that's okay. What matters is that you get back on track and continue making positive choices moving forward. Consistency builds healthy habits and creates a foundation for lasting results.

7. Self-Care and Stress Management

Taking care of your mental and emotional well-being is essential for making sustainable changes. Incorporate self-care practices that help you relax, manage stress, and improve overall mental health. This could include activities such as meditation, deep breathing exercises, spending time in nature, engaging in hobbies, or seeking support from a therapist or counselor. By addressing stress and nurturing your emotional well-being, you can better navigate challenges and maintain long-term lifestyle changes.

Maintaining A Healthy Weight

Maintaining a healthy weight is essential for overall well-being and can have numerous benefits for physical and mental health. It involves striking a balance between energy intake and energy expenditure to prevent weight gain or loss. Achieving weight maintenance requires adopting a sustainable lifestyle that includes healthy eating habits, regular physical activity, and other supportive strategies.

1. Healthy Eating Habits: A key component of weight maintenance is following a nutritious and balanced diet. Consider the following guidelines:

- **Portion Control**: Be mindful of portion sizes and avoid oversized servings. Use smaller plates and bowls to help control portions visually.

- **Choose Nutrient-Dense Foods**: Focus on

incorporating whole, unprocessed foods into your diet, including fruits, vegetables, whole grains, lean proteins, and healthy fats. These foods provide essential nutrients while keeping you satisfied.

- **Limit Added Sugars and Processed Foods**: Minimize the consumption of sugary beverages, snacks, and processed foods, as they are often high in calories and low in nutritional value.

2. Regular Physical Activity: Engaging in regular exercise is crucial for weight maintenance. Consider the following strategies:

- **Find Activities You Enjoy**: Choose physical activities that you genuinely enjoy, such as walking, swimming, dancing, or cycling. This will increase your motivation and make it easier to stick to a consistent exercise routine.

- **Set Realistic Goals**: Establish realistic and attainable goals for physical activity. Aim for at least 150 minutes of moderate-intensity aerobic exercise per week, along with strength training exercises two or more days a week.

- **Incorporate Physical Activity into Daily Life**: Look for opportunities to be more active throughout the day, such as taking the stairs instead of the elevator, walking or biking to nearby destinations, or incorporating short exercise breaks into your routine.

3. Mindful Eating: Practicing mindful eating can help

you maintain a healthy weight by fostering a better relationship with food and improving awareness of hunger and fullness cues. Consider the following techniques:

- **Slow Down**: Eat slowly and savor each bite. This allows your brain to register satiety and helps prevent overeating.

- **Pay Attention to Hunger and Fullness**: Tune in to your body's hunger and fullness signals. Eat when you're moderately hungry and stop eating when you feel comfortably satisfied.

- **Avoid Emotional Eating**: Distinguish between physical hunger and emotional triggers for eating. Find alternative ways to cope with stress, boredom, or other emotions instead of turning to food.

4. Regular Self-Monitoring: Regularly monitoring your weight, food intake, and physical activity can be an effective strategy for weight maintenance. Consider the following practices:

- **Weigh Yourself Regularly**: Weighing yourself weekly or monthly can help you stay aware of any fluctuations and take corrective action if necessary.

- **Keep a Food Journal**: Recording what you eat can increase your awareness of eating patterns and help identify areas for improvement.

- **Track Physical Activity**: Use a fitness tracker or smartphone app to monitor your daily physical activity and set goals for steps or active minutes.

5. Social Support: Having a support system can significantly impact your ability to maintain a healthy weight. Consider the following strategies:

- **Seek Support**: Join a weight loss or maintenance group, participate in online forums or social media groups, or enlist a friend or family member as an accountability partner.

- **Share Goals and Progress**: Communicate your weight maintenance goals with your support system, and regularly update them on your progress. This can help keep you motivated and provide a sense of accountability.

- **Celebrate Milestones**: Celebrate your achievements along the way, whether it's reaching a weight maintenance milestone or successfully sticking to your exercise routine. Rewarding yourself can help reinforce positive behaviors.

Strategies For Weight Maintenance In The Zone

The Zone Diet is a popular dietary approach that focuses on balancing macronutrients to achieve optimal hormonal balance and weight maintenance. The diet emphasizes consuming a specific ratio of carbohydrates, proteins, and fats to regulate insulin levels and promote steady energy levels. Here are some strategies for weight maintenance in The Zone:

1. Follow the 40-30-30 Ratio: The Zone Diet recommends consuming approximately 40% of calories from carbohydrates, 30% from proteins, and 30% from fats. This balanced macronutrient distribution helps stabilize blood sugar levels and control hunger.

- **Choose Low-Glycemic Carbohydrates**: Opt for carbohydrates that have a low glycemic index, such as whole grains, legumes, and non-starchy vegetables. These foods release glucose into the bloodstream more gradually, preventing rapid spikes in insulin levels.

- **Include Lean Proteins**: Incorporate lean protein sources like chicken, turkey, fish, tofu, and legumes into your meals. Protein is essential for maintaining muscle mass and promoting satiety.

- **Focus on Healthy Fats**: Consume sources of healthy fats, including avocados, nuts, seeds, olive oil, and fatty fish. These fats provide essential fatty acids and contribute to feelings of fullness.

2. Eat Balanced Meals: To maintain weight in The Zone, it's crucial to create balanced meals that adhere to the 40-30-30 ratio. Here's how you can structure your meals:

- **Divide Your Plate**: Mentally divide your plate into three equal sections. Fill one-third with a lean protein source, another third with low-glycemic carbohydrates, and the remaining third with healthy fats and non-starchy vegetables.

- **Control Portion Sizes**: Be mindful of portion sizes to maintain the appropriate balance of macronutrients. Use measuring cups or a food scale initially to ensure you're accurately portioning your food.

- **Include Fiber-Rich Foods**: Incorporate fiber-rich foods like fruits, vegetables, and whole grains to promote satiety and support digestive health.

3. Regularly Space Out Meals and Snacks: The Zone Diet recommends eating smaller, frequent meals and snacks throughout the day to maintain stable blood sugar levels and prevent energy crashes. This strategy can also help control hunger and cravings.

- **Eat Every 4-5 Hours**: Aim to eat a balanced meal or snack every 4-5 hours to keep your metabolism active and avoid extreme hunger.

- **Choose Healthy Snacks**: Opt for nutritious snacks that combine all three macronutrients. For example, pair a small handful of nuts with a piece of fruit or enjoy a Greek yogurt with some vegetables.

- **Listen to Your Body**: Pay attention to your body's hunger and fullness signals. Eat when you're moderately hungry and stop when you feel comfortably satisfied.

4. Stay Hydrated: Adequate hydration is crucial for overall health and weight maintenance. Make sure to drink enough water throughout the day to support proper bodily functions and promote satiety.

- **Drink Water with Meals**: Sip water during meals

to help fill you up and prevent overeating.

- **Limit Sugary Beverages**: Avoid or minimize the consumption of sugary drinks like soda, juice, and sweetened beverages. These drinks can add unnecessary calories and spike insulin levels.

5. Be Consistent and Flexible: Consistency is key when it comes to maintaining weight in The Zone. However, it's also essential to be flexible and make adjustments based on your individual needs and lifestyle.

- **Personalize the Ratio**: While the 40-30-30 ratio is a guideline, you can adjust it slightly to fit your preferences and needs. Some individuals may find a slightly higher protein intake more beneficial, while others may prefer a slightly higher carbohydrate intake. It's important to find the right balance that works for your body and supports your weight maintenance goals.

- **Stay Mindful of Portions**: Even within the recommended macronutrient ratios, portion control is essential. Be mindful of portion sizes and avoid overeating, even if the foods fit within the Zone parameters.

- **Make Healthy Food Choices**: While The Zone Diet doesn't restrict specific foods, it's important to prioritize nutrient-dense, whole foods. Choose lean proteins, complex carbohydrates, and healthy fats to support overall health and weight maintenance.

- **Listen to Your Body**: Pay attention to how different foods make you feel. Each person may have unique responses to certain foods, so listen to your body's cues and make adjustments as needed.

- **Adapt to Lifestyle Changes**: The Zone Diet can be adapted to various lifestyles, such as vegetarian or vegan diets. Focus on incorporating plant-based sources of protein and healthy fats while still adhering to the balanced macronutrient ratios.

- **Seek Professional Guidance**: If you're new to The Zone Diet or have specific health concerns, it's advisable to consult a registered dietitian or healthcare professional. They can provide personalized guidance and support to help you maintain a healthy weight effectively.

Remember that weight maintenance is a long-term commitment and requires sustainable lifestyle changes. The Zone Diet, with its focus on balanced macronutrient ratios, can be a helpful approach for weight maintenance. However, it's essential to listen to your body, make adjustments as needed, and prioritize overall health and well-being alongside weight management.

Recognizing And Preventing Weight Regain

Weight regain can be a common challenge for individuals who have previously lost weight. Sustaining long-term weight loss requires ongoing effort and adopting strategies to prevent relapse. Here are some tips to recognize and prevent weight regain:

1. Monitor Your Weight: Regularly monitoring your weight can help you catch any small increases early on before they become significant. Weigh yourself at consistent intervals and keep track of any changes. If you notice a gradual but consistent increase, it's time to take action.

2. Recognize Triggers and Emotional Eating: Identify the triggers that may lead to overeating or emotional eating. Stress, boredom, or certain social situations can contribute to mindless eating. Developing alternative coping strategies like exercise, meditation, or engaging in hobbies can help prevent weight regain.

3. Maintain a Support System: Surround yourself with a supportive network of friends, family, or even online communities that share your weight maintenance goals. Sharing your struggles, triumphs, and concerns can provide encouragement and accountability.

4. Establish Healthy Habits: Focus on adopting healthy habits that support weight maintenance. This includes regular physical activity, mindful eating, adequate sleep, and stress management. Consistency in these habits can help prevent weight regain.

5. Set Realistic Goals: Avoid setting unrealistic weight goals that may lead to frustration or a sense of failure. Instead, focus on maintaining a healthy weight range that is sustainable and achievable. Celebrate non-scale victories such as improved energy levels, increased fitness, or better overall health.

6. Practice Mindful Eating: Mindful eating involves paying attention to your body's hunger and fullness cues, as well as savoring each bite. Eating slowly, chewing thoroughly, and being fully present during meals can help prevent overeating and promote satisfaction.

7. Stay Active: Regular physical activity is crucial for weight maintenance. Engage in activities that you enjoy and make them a part of your daily routine. Find ways to incorporate movement into your day, such as walking, biking, or taking the stairs.

Enjoying The Benefits Of Increased Energy

Having ample energy throughout the day is crucial for leading a productive and fulfilling life. When we have high energy levels, we feel motivated, focused, and capable of taking on challenges. Here are some strategies to help you enjoy the benefits of increased energy:

1. Prioritize Sleep: Adequate sleep is the foundation for maintaining high energy levels. Aim for 7-9 hours of quality sleep each night. Establish a consistent sleep schedule and create a relaxing bedtime routine to ensure a restful night's sleep.

2. Stay Hydrated: Dehydration can lead to fatigue and low energy levels. Make it a habit to drink enough water throughout the day. Carry a reusable water bottle with you and set reminders if necessary.

3. Nourish Your Body: A balanced diet plays a vital role in sustaining energy levels. Consume a variety of nutrient-rich foods, including fruits, vegetables, whole grains, lean proteins, and healthy fats. Avoid excessive sugar and processed foods, as they can cause energy crashes.

4. Regular Exercise: Engaging in regular physical activity boosts energy levels by improving circulation, increasing oxygen flow, and releasing endorphins. Find activities you enjoy and incorporate them into your routine, whether it's walking, jogging, dancing, or playing sports.

5. Manage Stress: Chronic stress can drain your energy reserves. Practice stress management techniques like deep breathing, meditation, yoga, or engaging in hobbies you find relaxing. Take breaks throughout the day to recharge and reset your mind.

6. Optimize Your Environment: Surround yourself with an environment that promotes energy and vitality. Keep your workspace clean and organized, let in natural light, and add plants for a refreshing ambiance. Use uplifting scents or listen to energizing music to enhance your mood.

7. Limit Caffeine: While caffeine can provide a temporary energy boost, excessive consumption can disrupt sleep patterns and lead to energy crashes. Consume caffeine in moderation and avoid it close to bedtime.

8. Practice Mindfulness: Mindfulness can help you connect with the present moment, increase self-awareness, and conserve energy. Engage in mindfulness practices such as meditation, mindful eating, or simply taking a few minutes to pause and breathe deeply.

By implementing these strategies, you can enjoy the benefits of increased energy in your daily life. Remember that energy levels fluctuate throughout the day, so it's essential to listen to your body and give it the care and support it needs.

Tips For Sustaining Energy Levels Throughout The Day

Maintaining consistent energy levels throughout the day is crucial for productivity and well-being. When our energy dips, it becomes challenging to focus, stay motivated, and accomplish our goals. Here are some tips to help you sustain energy levels throughout the day:

1. Start with a Nutritious Breakfast: A healthy breakfast fuels your body and provides the energy you need to kick-start your day. Include a mix of complex carbohydrates, protein, and healthy fats in your morning meal. Whole-grain cereals, eggs, yogurt, and fruits are excellent choices.

2. Have Regular, Balanced Meals: Avoid skipping meals as it can lead to energy crashes. Instead, aim for regular, balanced meals and snacks throughout the day. Include a combination of protein, complex carbohydrates, and healthy fats to maintain steady energy levels.

3. Snack Smart: Choose nutrient-dense snacks that provide sustained energy. Opt for options like nuts, seeds, Greek yogurt, hummus with vegetables, or a piece of fruit with nut butter. Avoid sugary snacks that can cause energy spikes and subsequent crashes.

4. Stay Active: Physical activity is not only essential for overall health but also for sustaining energy levels. Take short breaks during the day to stretch, walk around, or engage in light exercise. Moving your body helps increase blood flow and oxygenation, boosting energy levels and reducing fatigue.

5. Stay Hydrated: Dehydration can contribute to feelings of fatigue. Make sure to drink enough water throughout the day to stay hydrated. Keep a water bottle handy and sip water regularly, even if you don't feel thirsty.

6. Practice Mindful Eating: Pay attention to how you eat. Slow down and savor your meals, chewing thoroughly and being mindful of the flavors and textures. Eating mindfully helps improve digestion and allows you to fully enjoy and benefit from the energy-boosting properties of your food.

7. Break Up Your Tasks: Long periods of focused work can be mentally draining and lead to decreased energy levels. Break up your tasks into manageable chunks and take short breaks in between. This allows your mind to recharge and helps maintain your energy throughout the day.

8. Get Fresh Air and Natural Light: Spending time outdoors and exposing yourself to natural light can have a positive impact on your energy levels. Take short breaks to go outside, whether it's for a walk, to sit in a park, or simply to enjoy the sunlight. Fresh air and natural light can help invigorate both your body and mind.

9. Prioritize Stress Management: Stress can deplete your energy reserves. Find healthy ways to manage stress, such as practicing relaxation techniques, engaging in hobbies, or seeking support from friends, family, or a professional. By reducing stress, you can maintain better energy levels throughout the day.

10. Get Sufficient Rest: In addition to a good night's sleep, it's essential to take regular breaks and allow yourself moments of rest throughout the day. This could include short power naps, moments of meditation or deep relaxation, or simply taking a few minutes to close your eyes and breathe deeply. Resting helps recharge your body and mind, promoting sustained energy levels.

11. Prioritize Tasks Strategically: Consider your energy levels and natural rhythms when scheduling your tasks. If possible, tackle your most challenging or mentally demanding tasks during your peak energy periods. Reserve less demanding tasks for when your energy naturally dips. By aligning your tasks with your energy levels, you can optimize your productivity and maintain better energy throughout the day.

Remember, everyone's energy levels fluctuate, so it's essential to listen to your body and adapt these tips to suit your individual needs. Experiment with different strategies and find what works best for you to sustain energy levels and maximize your productivity and well-being throughout the day.

CONCLUSION

Recap Of Key Points From The Ebook

In this section, we will recap some of the key points discussed in the eBook, highlighting the main concepts and ideas that can help readers on their journey towards achieving their goals.

1. Understanding the Zone: The eBook emphasized the importance of understanding the concept of "the Zone" and its relevance to personal growth and success. The Zone refers to a state of optimal performance and productivity where individuals are fully engaged in their tasks and experience a sense of flow. It is a mental state characterized by focus, clarity, and heightened performance.

2. Identifying Goals: The eBook emphasized the significance of setting clear and specific goals. By defining what you want to achieve, you can align your actions and efforts towards reaching those goals. It is crucial to set both short-term and long-term goals that are challenging yet attainable, providing a sense of direction and purpose.

3. Time Management: Effective time management is a vital aspect of maximizing productivity and achieving goals. The eBook discussed various strategies to manage time efficiently, such as prioritizing tasks, breaking them down into smaller, manageable steps, and eliminating distractions. By organizing and optimizing your time, you can make the most of each day and move closer to your objectives.

4. Building a Supportive Environment: Surrounding yourself with a supportive environment was highlighted as a key factor in sustaining motivation and achieving success. The eBook emphasized the importance of seeking encouragement, support, and accountability from like-minded individuals or mentors who can provide guidance and motivation along the way.

5. Overcoming Obstacles: The eBook acknowledged that challenges and setbacks are inevitable on any journey. It encouraged readers to adopt a growth mindset and view obstacles as opportunities for learning and growth. By embracing resilience and perseverance, individuals can navigate through difficulties and continue progressing towards their goals.

6. Celebrating Milestones: Recognizing and celebrating milestones along the way was emphasized as a way to maintain motivation and momentum. By acknowledging and rewarding yourself for the progress made, you can stay encouraged and inspired to keep moving forward on your Zone journey.

Encouragement And Motivation For Readers

To Start Their Zone Journey

Embarking on a Zone journey can be both exciting and daunting. Therefore, it is crucial to provide readers with the necessary encouragement and motivation to begin their own transformative journey. Here are a few key points to inspire readers to take that first step:

1. Believe in Yourself: Building self-belief is essential when starting any journey. Remind readers that they possess unique talents, abilities, and strengths that can be harnessed to achieve their goals. Encourage them to have faith in their potential and the impact they can make.

2. Start Small: Starting small can alleviate feelings of overwhelm and make the journey more manageable. Encourage readers to take the first step, no matter how small, and gradually build momentum. Each small success will create a positive feedback loop, further fueling motivation.

3. Embrace Imperfection: Perfectionism can hinder progress and discourage individuals from even beginning their journey. Encourage readers to embrace imperfection and focus on progress rather than striving for flawless execution. Remind them that setbacks and mistakes are natural and can be valuable learning experiences.

4. Find Inspiration: Inspire readers to seek out stories of others who have embarked on similar journeys and achieved success. Sharing real-life examples and case studies can motivate readers by demonstrating that their goals are attainable with effort and determination.

5. Visualize Success: Encourage readers to visualize their success and the fulfillment they will experience upon reaching their goals. Visualization techniques can help individuals stay focused, maintain motivation, and overcome obstacles along the way.

Final Thoughts And Next Steps For Achieving Their Goals

As readers conclude their reading of the eBook and embark on their Zone journey, it is important to provide them with final thoughts and guidance on the next steps they can take to achieve their goals. Here are some key points to consider:

1. Reflect on Insights: Encourage readers to take some time to reflect on the insights and knowledge gained from the eBook. They can do this by journaling or engaging in introspective activities. Reflection allows them to internalize the concepts and personalize them according to their unique circumstances and aspirations.

2. Set Clear Actionable Goals: Remind readers to revisit their goals and ensure they are clear, specific, and actionable. Encourage them to write down their goals and create a timeline or action plan to guide their progress. Breaking down bigger goals into smaller milestones can make them more attainable and provide a sense of accomplishment along the way.

3. Develop Daily Habits: Emphasize the importance of developing positive daily habits that align with their goals. Encourage readers to identify habits that will contribute to their growth and success, such as practicing mindfulness, setting aside dedicated time for skill development, or maintaining a consistent exercise routine. Consistency in these habits will pave the way for long-term progress.

4. Seek Accountability: Suggest that readers find an accountability partner or join a supportive community where they can share their goals and progress. Having someone to hold them accountable can significantly increase their motivation and commitment to achieving their goals. Online forums, social media groups, or local meetups can provide valuable support and encouragement.

5. Embrace Continuous Learning: Remind readers that learning is a lifelong journey. Encourage them to seek out opportunities for continuous learning and personal development. This could involve reading books, attending seminars, taking online courses, or connecting with mentors who can provide guidance and wisdom.

6. Stay Resilient and Flexible: Remind readers that the journey towards their goals may not always be smooth. Encourage them to stay resilient and adaptable in the face of challenges and setbacks. Remind them that setbacks are temporary and can be valuable learning experiences.

Encourage them to stay committed to their goals and adjust their strategies when necessary.

www.ingramcontent.com/pod-product-compliance
Lightning Source LLC
Chambersburg PA
CBHW050730260726
48661CB00001B/157